The Informed Practice Nurse

Edited by
MARILYN EDWARDS

Specialist Practitioner, General Practice Nursing,
Bilbrook Medical Centre, Staffordshire

W

WHURR PUBLISHERS

LONDON

© 1999 Whurr Publishers
First published 1999 by
Whurr Publishers Ltd
19b Compton Terrace, London N1 2UN, England

British Library Cataloguing in Publication Data
A catalogue record for this book is available from the
British Library.

ISBN: 1 86156 096 6

Printed and bound in the UK by Athenaeum Press Ltd,
Gateshead, Tyne & Wear

Contents

Contributors

Carol Atton BSc(Hons), SRD Community Disorders Service Manager, Black Country Mental Health NHS Trust, Sandwell.

Mandy Beaumont RGN Clinical Nurse Specialist, Infection Control, South Staffs Health Authority.

Wendy Cieslik RGN, DipPHS Practice Nurse, Bilbrook Medical Centre, Bilbrook, Staffordshire.

Jean Crutchley RGN, BSc(Hons), DipPHS, PNCert Clinical Nurse Specialist, Respiratory Care, New Cross Hospital, Wolverhampton.

Marilyn Edwards SRN, BSc(Hons), DipPHS, FEATC, PNCert, SchNCert Specialist Practitioner, General Practice Nursing, Bilbrook Medical Centre, Bilbrook, Staffordshire.

Diana Forster MSc, BA(Hons), RGN, RM, RHV, RHVT, RNT Formerly Head of Health Studies, University of North London; currently freelance writer and consultant in health and health psychology.

Helen Jenkinson RGN, DPSN Clinical Nurse Specialist, Infection Control, South Staffs Health Authority.

Susan Jones BSc, SRD Paediatric Dietician, New Cross Hospital, Wolverhampton.

Gudrun Limbrick BA(Hons). Freelance writer, founder of Lesbian Health Group, LesBeWell.

Cath Molineux RGN, BSc(Hons), OND, OHNC Specialist Practitioner, General Practice Nursing, Stepping Stones Medical Practice, Dudley, West Midlands.

Georgina Paget BSc(Hons), RGN, OND(Hons) Clinical Nurse Specialist (HIV/AIDS), First Community Health NHS Trust, South Staffordshire.

Diane Pannell SRN, SCM, DipMid, HECert Formerly Community Midwife, Bromsgrove and Redditch.

Joy Rainey MSc, BSc, DipSN, RGN, DN Clinical Nurse Specialist, Wound Care, Wolverhampton Health Authority.

Pat Tweed SRN, MSc, BSc(Hons), FEATC, CertPN(Keele), FPCert Specialist Practitioner, General Practice Nursing, Practice Nurse Co-ordinator, Gnosall, Staffordshire.

Glen Turp RGN Royal College of Nursing Regional Officer.

Preface

Practice nursing has become an increasingly popular speciality within primary health care in recent years. As general practitioners' workload increases, more and more doctors are allowing their nursing colleagues a higher level of autonomy to plan, implement and assess certain areas of patient care, in an attempt to achieve ever-changing government objectives. This would have been unheard of in the 'nurse-as-a-handmaiden' era and demonstrates the increasingly important role of the nursing profession in providing primary care.

The purpose of this book is to increase nurses' awareness of some of the key issues within general practice that may be causing concern or confusion, placing them in context within the nurse's changing role. Although the book is aimed primarily at practice nurses, the issues addressed are relevant to nurses of all disciplines working within general practice.

Specialists have contributed key topics that are currently not addressed in practice nursing textbooks but are increasingly relevant in primary care. These include the practice nurse's role in sexual health, pre-conceptual care and dietetics. Nurses must be willing to liaise with other health-related disciplines if they wish to achieve a high level of patient care.

It is hoped that issues raised within this book will stimulate the reader to undertake research or study to improve patient care within general practice.

Marilyn Edwards
January 1999

Introduction

This book has been planned to meet the needs of practice nurses, although many issues relate to other community nurses. Examples of real or hypothesized practice, with recommendations for implementing quality care, relate specifically to general practice. The reader will probably be able to relate other examples to fit individual topics.

Most of the chapters are sub-divided into specific subject areas. For example, the chapter on *Women's Health* is sub-divided to include pre-menstrual syndrome, promoting continence and the health needs of lesbians. This structuring allows ease of access to a specific topic.

Nursing ethics underpins all patient care and is essential to protect both nurses and patients. Personal and professional accountability and patient autonomy, which are integral to all aspect of patient care, are stressed throughout the book and should stay in the forefront of the reader's mind.

Although the book is not a clinical handbook, wound management is included to demonstrate how all the introductory chapters relate to patient care. The reader can transfer these issues to any other areas of practice or community nursing. Some areas may appear unnecessary to some readers as 'everyone knows that', but, from the editor's experience, there are practising nurses who do not follow recommended guidelines.

'Health Improvement Programmes' are the buzz words of 1999. Primary care groups will be expected to assess locality needs and plan health care accordingly. The reader is given guidelines on assessing needs and profiling in Chapter 4. Multidisciplinary consultation is essential to assess needs fully. When profiles are used in conjunction with quality assurance, nurses are in a strong position to influence primary care group policy, either directly, or indirectly, though a spokesperson. Doctors will need the support of nurses to provide the evidence for clinical governance.

Evidence-based information is crucial to support nursing practice and will be found throughout the text. There is inevitably some overlap between chapters because topics cannot be compartmentalized. This overlap will reinforce relevant issues. The content of the book is explained through a brief précis of the rationale for, and content of, each chapter. A comprehensive index will allow the reader to access specific points.

It is hoped that issues raised in this book will encourage nurses at all levels to question their practice where necessary and to use evidence-based knowledge to negotiate appropriate care for their patients.

Quality nursing is independent of the political climate with its constant change of health policy; this has deliberately been omitted from the text.

Chapter 1
Ethics

Pat Tweed, Cath Molineux and Marilyn Edwards

The word 'ethical' relates to morals, the science of ethics or professional standards of conduct (Chambers Dictionary, 1993). This
morality is influenced by genetics, socialization, education and life
events. The study of ethics helps one to consider what kinds of thing
are good or bad and how to decide whether actions are right or
wrong.

The role of codes of practice in ethical decision-making is
discussed in this chapter using examples from general practice. The
reader will recognize many of the examples cited in the chapter and
will probably be able to describe many more.

Doctors and nurses may sometimes forget the rights of patients in
the rush to 'get the job done', meet targets and appear efficient. This
is an area that nurses can readily address and possibly share with
their primary health care team colleagues. Informed consent, for
both adults and minors, is essential if patients are to be involved in
their care and be autonomous.

The issues discussed within this chapter are pertinent to all areas
of nursing care and are referred to throughout the book.

Codes of practice: how effective are they in ethical decision-making?

In order to assess the effectiveness of codes of practice in making
ethical decisions in nursing, one first needs to consider what is meant
by an 'ethical decision'. This section examines the codes of practice
for nurses, following a brief description of ethical principles. The
Code of Professional Conduct (UKCC, 1992a) will be referred to as
'the Code', the principles of which may conflict with issues relating

to power and authority in the primary health care setting. The document 'Scope of Professional Practice' (UKCC, 1992b) will be referred to as 'Scope'. Guidance available to assist ethical decision-making in confidentiality, and advertising and sponsorship within general practice, will be addressed.

Ethical philosophies and theories

The two main philosophies of ethical reasoning, utilitarianism and deontology, have almost diametrically opposed prime principles (Seedhouse, 1988). Utilitarianism was propounded by John Stuart Mill and Jeremy Bentham, who believed that the ends justify the means and that the right action is the one which offers the greatest good to the greatest number. Deontology is the theory associated with Immanuel Kant. It is based on duty and respect for the individual, who must be treated as an end in himself and never as a means to an end. It is the action itself that is right or wrong; the consequences are less important.

When faced with a moral dilemma, 'with two alternative choices, neither of which seems a satisfactory solution to the problem' (Campbell, cited in Jones, 1994), a decision has to be made based on one's own moral principles and what each person believes to be right. The rules that guide thinking are known as ethical principles. Beneficence and non-maleficence, actively doing good and the avoidance of harm, are two principles often described by ethical philosophers and writers. Beneficence is said by Seedhouse to unite deontology and utilitarianism:

> we do not seek to maximise good over evil simply because the consequences are better for most people, but because we have a duty to do good and prevent harm. (Seedhouse, 1988, p. 136)

In his text on ethical theory and practice, Thiroux (1980) outlines five ethical principles that he considers to be applicable to all spheres of life (Box 1.1).

Box 1.1: Ethical principles applicable to all spheres of life

- The value of life and respect for persons
- Goodness or rightness
- Justice or fairness
- Truth-telling or honesty
- Individual freedom or autonomy

The function of codes

The three functions of professional codes identified by Burnard and Chapman (1988) are ethical, political and disciplinary. This section will concentrate mainly on the first of these, although the impact of the other two will be clearly shown.

The Code sets out the professional accountability of each registered nurse, midwife and health visitor to the patient or client, to the health care team and to society as a whole. Pyne (1988) describes the Code as 'a statement to the profession of the primacy of the patients' interest', whilst Chadwick and Tadd (1992) describe it as a 'stimulus to moral thinking' rather than a code of ethics.

Although the Code may have considerable influence over a nurse's resolution of ethical dilemmas, each situation for each person is unique and is only a guide to decision-making. A code may stress the most important considerations that should influence a decision, but a nurse cannot turn to the Code and expect it to provide a moral answer to an ethical problem, 'for nurses, like other competent adults, have the capacity for autonomy and making moral choices and they do not leave this behind when they go on duty' (Chadwick and Tadd, 1992).

Codes of practice are meant to reassure members of the public about the quality of the professional service, as well as enhancing the public image of the individual practitioner. The Code, applicable to all nurses, midwives and health visitors, those in management posts and those in clinical situations, is 'designed to result in action' (Pyne, 1988). It can be used to fight for improvements in standards, although this is not always an easy path to take, as will be seen later.

Professional codes also play a part in supporting the status of a profession. A code of conduct has been said to be one of the defining characteristics of a profession (Jaggar, quoted in Chadwick and Tadd, 1992). The implication is that those within the group can be trusted to regulate their members and, if necessary, discipline them if they fail to uphold the high standards of the code.

The United Kingdom Central Council for Nursing, Midwifery and Health Visiting (UKCC) has legal status and authority, under the Nurses, Midwives and Health Visitors Act of 1979, to prepare rules that carry the weight of law. However, the Code is issued for guidance and advice, laying a moral responsibility rather than a statutory duty, on members of the profession (Young, 1989). The Code can be used by a nurse to measure her own conduct, in the knowledge that the requirements of the Code are used by the UKCC as 'a backcloth against which allegations of misconduct are now judged' (Pyne, 1988). Failure to comply with these may result in nurses losing their registration.

The Code of Professional Conduct is therefore a guide, a political statement and a means of regulating the profession.

The emphasis of the Code

The Code commits each individual nurse, midwife and health visitor to safeguard and promote the interests of both society and individual patients and clients. It also requires that each 'shall act at all times in such a manner as to justify public trust and confidence and to uphold and enhance the good standing and reputation of the professions' (UKCC, 1992a). In order for the nurse to fulfil these requirements, emphasis is placed on four main areas: knowledge, skill, responsibility and accountability. The principles of the Scope of Professional Practice (UKCC, 1992b) are based upon these aspects.

Bergman (1981) listed four preconditions to accountability, which were almost the same as the areas defined by the Code, but also included the need for authority (Figure 1.1).

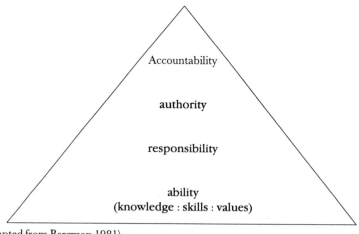

(adapted from Bergman 1981)

Figure 1.1: Preconditions to accountability.

Knowledge and skill

The Code places upon the practitioner the continuing responsibility to maintain and develop her knowledge, skill and competence through self-assessment and the production of a personal portfolio. Clauses 3 and 4 of the Code state clearly that each nurse must acknowledge personal limits of knowledge and skill and take steps to remedy any relevant deficits in order to meet the needs of patients and clients, a reflection of Thiroux's principle of honesty.

The Code does not say what each nurse must learn, but acts as a guide. A nurse, faced with the dilemma of being asked or instructed to carry out a procedure that she does not feel fully competent to do has the support of clear principles upon which to act.

The perception of competence can differ between the nurse and the employer (Jones, 1996, p. 83). This is a common situation in general practice, in which the old medical adage of 'see one, do one, teach one' is often quoted. The ethical principles involved here are non-maleficence, the primacy of the patients' interest (respect for persons) and the justification of public trust. 'Casual acceptance of duties or responsibilities is dangerous practice and work should not be taken on, until the individual nurse feels safe and secure in her own performance' (Castledine, 1992).

Responsibility and accountability

Responsibility for tasks or areas of patient care is given to an individual practitioner. Accountability is the acceptance of that responsibility and the willingness to explain one's actions and to receive credit or blame for the results of those actions (Evans, 1993). One can be responsible but not accountable, although one cannot be accountable without being responsible (Young, 1989). A registered nurse, midwife or health visitor is accountable to the client, the profession, the law and the employer (Figure 1.2).

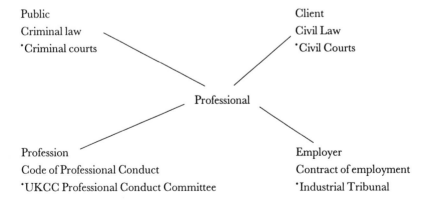

Figure 1.2: Areas of professional accountability, indicating the groups to whom the registered nurse is accountable, the basis of that accountability and the authority empowered to judge the actions of the nurse in each area.

In the rush to extend the scope of nursing practice into new areas, the Scope emphasizes that existing professional care must not be compromised or fragmented (Clause 9.4). Practice nurses are developing their role in primary health care, sometimes by taking over work that was previously seen as the province of the doctor. Castledine (1992) warns that medical knowledge and skills, no matter how relevant to medical practice and health care, are no substitutes for the development of nursing knowledge and skills. The role of the nurse should develop in response to patient need and through experience gained by post-basic education (Carlisle, 1992).

In general practice, this development has resulted in nurses taking the lead in caring for people with chronic conditions such as asthma and diabetes. This work requires both medical knowledge and nursing skills of education, health promotion and counselling. Such a model of practice, when pursued, facilitates patient autonomy through participation in the decision-making process, an expression of accountability highlighted by the Code (Clause 5) and supported by Evans (1993). However, it is all too easy to take on the medical model of treatment and cure, accepting the delegation of a task, such as the application of cryocautery, from a doctor (Jones, 1996, p. 125). Nursing skills can be soon forgotten in the excitement and interest of new technology.

The degree of accountability within a particular situation must surely be linked to the measure of authority held by the individual as, without that authority, one is not free to make an ethical decision regarding a problem (Tadd, 1994). The Code does not mention this concept in relation to accountability but insists that all practitioners are equally accountable.

Issues of power and authority

In a work situation, conflict may arise between the humanist values of the Code and the authoritarian values of the organization. Tschudin (1994a) writes that safeguarding and promoting the interests of patients and clients may or may not mean following instructions. Challenging authority is never easy, as shown by the experience of Graham Pink, but many other nurses have stood up for their clients, as recounted in the 'Value of Nursing' (RCN, 1992), with happier results.

Challenging action could be considered as advocacy on behalf of a patient, an advocate being defined as 'one who pleads the cause of another' (Chambers Dictionary, 1993). This is a positive, constructive activity recommended as a role for nursing by the UKCC (1989), particularly where a person is incapable of giving informed consent. The issue of informed consent will be addressed later in this chapter.

The nurse–doctor relationship

In general practice, the doctor may have been used to making all decisions regarding the care of his patients and may attempt to impose his authority over the work or decisions of other members of the team, work in which he has no particular training or skill. Chadwick and Tadd (1992) argue that, where issues are of an ethical nature, the doctor has no particular expertise and should not hold power. The nurse has a responsibility to point out poor practice, to explain current thinking and, if necessary, to refuse to take part in a procedure; refusing, for example, to assist in minor surgery with unsterile instruments, or to apply a dressing that could prejudice wound healing and cause harm.

The doctor's authority in medical matters is legitimate only if he performs correctly. The nurse must intervene if she knows or suspects it to be wrong (Chadwick and Tadd, 1992). In acting to safe-guard the well-being of a patient (Clause 1), the nurse must be aware that, although this may mean acting as the patient's advocate, she must not place herself outside other sections of the law by refusing to co-operate with treatment that the doctor has prescribed (Young, 1989, p. 206).

If the problem were of a serious nature, the nurse might feel it necessary, in order to protect the patient (Clause 11), to report the matter to a higher authority. This will probably be the health author-ity through the nurse adviser since practice nurses do not usually have the support of a more senior nurse in the workplace. Jones (1996, p. 146) reports an incident that, although badly handled in many ways, upheld the ethical principle of non-maleficence and achieved a satisfactory outcome for future patients. This action may be seen by many as a breach of health care team loyalties, and, combined with a public dislike of tale-telling, could result in a poss-ible loss of employment and reputation.

The probable harm, in the form of damage to team relationships, or public mistrust should it become more widely known, must be weighed against the benefit to patient care. Publicizing a problem in this way may only make it more difficult for others to complain in the future. The profession of nursing offers little in the way of support to those nurses who publicly exercise their accountability to the public by making official their concern about poor practice (Tadd, 1994).

Truth and trust

Trust has to be earned; it places obligations upon the individual nurse, not least of which is honesty. Truth-telling is not mentioned in the Code, although the more recent UKCC guidelines (1996) do refer to this principle in relation to the giving of information. Failure to be honest with a patient and answer questions relating, for example, to an incurable disease, because of a moral decision made by medical staff and/or relatives, conflicts with obligations relating to competency, consent and right to information. This is likely to destroy the relationship of trust and confidence. Chadwick and Tadd (1992) quote a survey in which 94% of patients questioned wanted to be told if they were dying, yet 80% of family doctors would lie to patients. This was often because the doctor did not know how to break the news. The responsibility to provide information rests with the practitioner, and 'if something less than the whole truth is told, it should never be because the practitioner is unable to cope with the effects of telling the truth' (UKCC, 1989).

Abuse of the individual practitioner

Nurses have always accepted the need to do their best in difficult circumstances, even to the extent of pretending that they can cope when they clearly cannot (Pyne, 1994). The Code states that 'the interest of the patient must always take precedence', but is this the short- or long-term interest? The short-term harm must be weighed against the possible long-term benefit. Nursing management has a responsibility to draw attention to an inadequacy of resources when an unacceptable workload is placed on individual practitioners (Clauses 12 and 13). Pyne (1992) urges nurses to support each other in the interests of the client, but many practice nurses still work alone, so that the need for a system of peer support, with a route to senior nurses within the health authority, is vital. Such support was largely lacking within the hospital setting, as demonstrated in the case of Graham Pink, the charge nurse who lost his job after upholding the Code by reporting a shortage of trained staff and his fears for patient care.

The ethical principle of 'respect for persons' applies to collea, as well as to clients (Tschudin, 1994b). The abusive treatment of in viduals who complain was highlighted by Beardshaw (1981) and years later by Tadd (1991), showing that little had changed. During the early 1990s, the NHS actively suppressed the right of employees to 'blow the whistle' on poor practice, through 'gagging clauses' in contracts, but a change in government has promised to ensure the end of this practice (Milburn, 1997, p. 13).

Confidentiality

Confidentiality, in the clinical setting, implies respect for information about a patient or client that has been given in trust. This information will not be passed to other people without the consent of the patient or client, except where disclosure is required by law or by the order of a court, or is necessary in the public interest (Clause 10). The Code stresses that breaches of confidentiality should be regarded as exceptional:

> Organisations which employ professional staff who make records are the legal owners of these records, but that does not give anyone in that organisation the legal right of access to the information in those records. (UKCC, 1996, p. 28)

Where shared records are used, the author of any particular entry must satisfy himself that other people with access to that shared record will respect the confidentiality of the information (UKCC, 1987). Shared records are becoming more common, but the above principle must always be borne in mind, for other professions, for example social workers, may hold a different view of 'the need to know' (Black, 1990).

Patient-held records involve the patient sharing in and having ownership of his own record. Asthma and diabetes are two of the conditions for which records may be taken by the patient to a variety of professionals for information to be recorded and shared, but the patient must be a partner in this, controlling the flow of information and not just transporting the card.

On occasions, patients may share with the nurse personal information that they do not want recorded or passed to a third person. They have a right to expect that their wishes will be complied with, for if they cannot rely on respect for confidences, they will be unlikely to seek help when they desperately need it.

There are, however, instances when acting in the interest of the patient may conflict with the interest of society; for example, when the information concerns the welfare of a third person who may be at risk, such as a child in a family where there is violence against another person.

The General Medical Council explains public interest disclosure by reference to the exposure of a patient or other person to a risk of death or serious harm (Korgaonkar and Tribe, 1994). The practitioner should discuss the matter fully with other practitioners and, if appropriate, consult with a professional organization without identifying the person concerned. When a decision is made to record or disclose the information without consent, the nurse must be prepared to justify that decision (UKCC, 1992a). Alternatively, if a decision is made not to disclose or record the information in the record, it must be recorded elsewhere along with the reasons for such action and be kept for future reference (UKCC, 1987).

The UKCC document on 'Confidentiality' (1987) warned of the danger of 'careless talk'. Sadly, this basic human failing is not mentioned in later documents. Discussion of a patient's problems with a colleague in a public place, such as in an office that is open to a waiting area, or on a telephone in reception, can cause confidential information to be released into the public domain and bring about complete loss of faith in the service. Even in areas that are reserved for staff, confidential details can be passed around over coffee so that information that a patient shared in confidence with one professional becomes public property.

The question of which members of the primary health care team need to have access to information about a specific patient needs to be asked on each separate occasion: there can be no overall right of access without a court order. Patients and clients must be made aware of the need for information to be shared, on occasions, with other health professionals, and of who those people are likely to be. The larger the team becomes, the greater the need for awareness of these issues.

Many general practices offer training facilities, so patients may find themselves confronted by a Project 2000 student or family planning student instead of the individual nurse whom they expected to see. Ideally, patient consent should be obtained prior to the person encountering the learner in order to give him a chance to request privacy if he so wishes. Even if there is no objection, it is important that the patient is allowed to control the flow of information. The requirements of the student must not take precedence over the need to seek consent.

Activity 1.1: Consider how your workplace, reception, treatment rooms, computer screens and telephones threaten the confidentiality of patient information. What changes could be made to protect confidentiality?

Advertising and sponsorship

The Code warns against the use of professional qualifications in the promotion of commercial products (Clause 16) 'in order not to compromise the independence of professional judgement on which patients and clients rely' (UKCC, 1996, p. 31). It is considered unacceptable for a nurse to wear a logo on a uniform, but how many boxes of tissues, pens, notepads or even appointment cards have a drug name printed on them?

A nurse may wish to recommend a blood glucose meter that she believes to be reliable in monitoring diabetes, or give out health promotion leaflets or information sponsored by a drug company. This could be considered manipulation by a commercial concern or may give the impression that the profession as a body recommends a product when other nurses might disagree (Chadwick and Tadd, 1992).

Nurses deal with people who are vulnerable and open to suggestion. Thus it is incumbent upon nurses to see that literature used has first been read, to ensure that the message is balanced and unbiased and does not directly promote a product or a company. It would be wise to discuss several makes of glucose meter, pointing out their advantages and disadvantages, and any independent evaluation, then allowing the patient to make his own choice.

Drug company sponsorship for study days and research projects is especially common in general practice. It is reasonable to assume that the valuable support of a company can lead to the advocacy of a particular product because of greater familiarity.

Activity 1.2: Consider the areas of patient care in which you influence the choice of treatment. Do the drug companies who make the products you choose most frequently also provide sponsored educational events for nurses? Do you think your judgement is swayed by commercial propaganda?

Summary

Orme and Maggs (1993) found that effective decision-making is an integral part of the clinical role of the practitioner. It often involves risk-taking within the parameters of the professional accountability placed upon each registered nurse by the UKCC Code of Conduct. Indeed, the Report of the Heathrow Debate (DoH, 1993, p. 308) reiterates a comment that 'nurses will not have arrived until they are sued'. It is hoped that this will not be the case.

The Code has been identified as a guide to making an appropriate response in a morally troubling situation. It is directed toward furthering the interests of patients, and through this comes the power of the nurse (Pyne, 1994). The use of knowledge and skill to serve the interest of the individual patient and society requires a willingness to empower those we serve through honesty, advocacy and the development of an environment within nursing in which those who take risks on behalf of patients are supported by senior colleagues. Within the areas of concern discussed, the development and application of a philosophy of care based on the Code would help to inform decision-making and provide a focus for professional practice. The Code will not provide an easy answer, but it may help us to find the right answer through 'trust rather than pretence and assertiveness rather than subservience' (Pyne, 1994).

Key points:

- Codes are meant to reassure members of the public with regard to the quality of a professional service.
- The Code lays a moral responsibility rather than a statutory duty on members of the profession.
- The Code makes the practitioner responsible for maintaining and developing her own knowledge, skill and competence.
- The question of who needs to have access to information about a specific patient needs to be asked on each separate occasion.

Issues of consent

The legal system in the UK requires consent from any patient or client who is about to undergo any treatment or surgical intervention. Without consent from the client, the nurse or doctor delivering the care may be in danger of being sued for assault and battery. The following text relates to adults, minors and persons with a learning disability.

What is consent?

Consent to any medical or surgical intervention is a legal arrangement based on the notion of a contract between two equal parties

(Alderson, 1995). There is some debate over whether equality exists between these two parties. The health professional would appear to have the upper hand by having greater knowledge of the procedure being undertaken. This may create barriers between the health professional and client in such a way that:

- the patient feels coerced into something against his will;
- some doctors claim that it is unfair to burden patients with technicalities they would not understand.

Although some clients may wish to take the submissive role and allow decisions to be made for them, this decision-making is not the role of the health professional. Information regarding the procedure must be imparted to the client, who is then enabled to make his own decision – informed consent. This issue will be discussed later.

Express and implied consent

Consent can be given in two ways: expressly or by implication. Express consent is usually in the form of writing, an example of which is the pre-operative consent form. Parents or guardians who attend with a child for vaccination will normally be expected to sign a consent form and often ask 'Do I have to sign anything?'

Nurses working within general practice usually encounter implied consent. If a client attends the surgery for treatment, this implies that he consents to the treatment, although a full explanation must be given beforehand. It would be assumed that a client who voluntarily attends a 'flu clinic' and proffers an arm for vaccination has given implied consent for the procedure.

Consent in English law

It is a basic rule of English law that no one has any right to touch another person without his consent. A nurse may not therefore do anything to clients without obtaining their agreement. The importance of this law is to ensure that clients understand and agree to the treatment suggested. Consent must be uncoerced and informed, and the benefit of any intervention must outweigh any harmful effects (Bird and White, 1995).

Exceptions to this law involve some aspects of nursing care. These include activities of nursing that assist the patient to do what he would normally do for himself, i.e. activities of daily living. Refusal of any assistance must be respected. This exception also permits the nurse to care for unconscious patients (Alderson, 1995), although a nurse working within general practice is unlikely to encounter this scenario.

Competence to consent

Chadwick and Tadd (1992) suggest that certain groups of people may not be able to give their consent for a medical or surgical procedure. Informed consent may be hindered by illness, stress, mental illness or a learning disability. If a person is mentally incapable of understanding the nature of the treatment, the consent form is invalid. It is therefore necessary for all health professionals to assess a client's mental competence before obtaining consent for treatment.

The Mental Health Act Code of Practice 1983, paragraph 15.10, states that certain criteria are necessary for a person to be able to consent to treatment (Box 1.2).

Box 1.2: The criteria necessary for a person to be able to consent (Mental Health Act 1993, para. 15.10)

The client:
1. understands what the treatment is and why he/she needs it
2. understands in broad terms the nature of the treatment
3. understands the benefits and risks
4. understands the consequences of not having the treatment
5. possesses the mental capacity to make a choice

If a client is unable to give consent owing to a psychological disorder, illness or stress, it is usually left to the relatives to shoulder the burden, although the final decision will lie with the doctor. A diagnosis of mental illness does not necessarily mean that the ability to give valid consent is affected.

Fullbrook (1994) argued that the question of a client's competence to consent to treatment is rarely raised unless there is an issue of non-compliance. For example, if a client refused life-saving surgery, his mental competence to make such a decision would be raised. However, if this same person consented to treatment, would his decision-making ability be questioned? Most probably not.

Fullbrook (1994) also states that the capacity to make a decision is judged in relation to the importance of the intervention. This scenario can be related to general practice. A client who, after consultation with his general practitioner, decides against a minor surgical procedure, would have his decision respected. If this same person refuses major surgery, his mental competence could be questioned. The reader may have cared for women with advanced breast cancer who chose not to have surgery, and may have found it difficult to accept this decision.

Competence to consent can therefore be linked to a question of conforming. An individual has a right to make his decisions, but mental competence may be questioned if the final decision fails to conform to society's expectations (Fullbrook, 1994). Standards may be either the norm for an individual or for society. Usually, when such a conflict arises, the final decision is made by the person with the most authority and knowledge.

It would appear that clients and their families in the late 1990s are now more informed regarding health care and patients' rights. The Patient's Charter (DoH, 1993) developed an increased awareness of a person's right to self-determination. There is an increasing expectation that decision-making should be both fully informed and collaborative. Health care professionals have come to recognize and respect the autonomy of individuals, moving away from prescriptive nursing care towards a negotiated contract of care.

Consent for clients with learning difficulties

Mentally compromised patients are said to be unable to, or not allowed to, exercise their autonomy to its fullest extent because the ability to make autonomous decisions must be competency based (Fullbrook, 1994). However, Fullbrook states that mental competence is not easily measured and may require expert analysis. This is a complex process, and in clinical practice the assessment of mental competence tends to be value judgements based on social and personal values (Hepworth, 1989).

Consent for clients with severe learning difficulties, the senile and those in a coma, who are all regarded as incompetent to give valid consent, is usually sought from a third party. Although relatives are often asked to make surrogate decisions on behalf of the patients, Fullbrook (1994) suggests that they may be mentally incompetent themselves owing to stress that may affect rational judgement.

Hanford (1993) raises ethical issues surrounding disability. She states that 'disability is rarely, if ever, given consideration in ethics teaching, even though autonomy is central to the concerns of the disabled'. This can relate to physical or mental disability. The sterilization of severely handicapped young women demonstrates the importance of ethical judgements in this client group: client A was made a ward of court and sterilized with the support of her mother, whereas the judge in a similar case in Canada would not agree to sterilize client B in these circumstances. Hanford raises concerns about the moral stance that professionals assume in ethical deliberations, which is central to any discussion on ethics and disability. Alternative methods of managing the sexuality of clients with a mental handicap are suggested. This is based on a 'caring' perspective that focuses on ethical care.

Nurses who care for clients with a learning disability may well have encountered the challenge of competence and consent. The three main areas of concern are immunization, contraception and cervical cytology. These are invasive procedures that may be difficult to explain in a language the client understands. Many of the clients who live in the community will have a key worker who has a deeper understanding of their client's mental ability. It may be necessary to defer a procedure until the key worker can obtain the necessary consent.

A person is more likely to give valid consent if the explanation is appropriate to the level of his assessed ability (Rumbold, 1993). Nurses should perhaps utilize the expertise of social workers or nurses trained in mental disability to ensure that clients with limited mental competence receive quality care, although issues of confidentiality are paramount.

Informed consent

The concept of informed consent has existed for many years within the medical profession. Cadoza in 1914 stated that 'Every human being of adult years and sound mind has a right to determine what shall be done with his body; and a surgeon who performs an operation without his patient's consent commits an assault for which he is liable for damages' (cited in Rumbold, 1993).

Informed consent has been defined as the patient's right to know what is entailed before any procedure is carried out (Chadwick and Tadd, 1992). This includes an explanation of any hazards or complications and the expected final outcome of treatment. Within general practice, it is the nurse's responsibility to ensure that the client is fully informed about any procedure, even when he has given implied consent by attending the surgery.

The client must be given all the relevant information in order for consent to be obtained. In England, there is no actual law that stipulates how much information is given, but it is the health professional's duty to ensure that there is no undue pressure or influence on the client. These issues emphasize the link between consent and autonomy in allowing individuals to be autonomous and permitted to make their own decisions regarding their health care.

Chadwick and Tadd (1992) argue that informed consent does not exist genuinely between professional and client as the client can never fully understand the information he is given. This reinforces the issue of an unequal contract between health professional and client. As mentioned before, stress and illness may influence the client's ability to make a rational decision even if all the information has been provided. It may be appropriate in some instances to defer a treatment until informed consent can be obtained.

Main principles of informed consent

Although some clients are unable to form an informed opinion, it must be remembered that everyone has the same rights; and the two main principles must be (Rumbold, 1993):

- Give people the respect due to any human being.
- Ensure that the person is protected from harm.

If a person is unable to give informed consent, 'it is considered good practice to discuss any proposed treatment with the next of kin' (NHSME, 1990), although the doctor does not have to obtain consent from the next of kin as the final decision in law rests with him.

Cultural issues

Regard must be given to the cultural backgrounds within the practice population when examining all the issues of informed consent in both adults and children. Difficulties with language can clearly have

---

Box 1.3: Examples of where language barriers may prevent the nurse obtaining informed consent

- Parents who do not speak or understand English, who are unable to give informed consent to a procedure for their child
- Administering vaccines, including influenza
- Prescribing diabetic medication and insulin
- Undertaking any bodily examination, including cervical smears
- Travel advice, including the choice of malaria prophylaxis

an impact when obtaining consent for treatment (Box 1.3). An interpreter is usually required for clients whose first language is not English. This may be a child or relative, which creates problems with sensitive issues and client confidentiality, although without an interpreter, the client is unable to give informed consent.

Minors and consent

Children are an important client group to be considered when examining issues of consent. Children are dependent on their parents or carers for their health and safety. Most parents look to health professionals to help them to make the right choices to ensure that their children grow up with healthy lives. It is customary in the UK to obtain the consent of a parent or guardian before carrying out treatment on a minor, although there is no statute law stating that a child cannot give consent to, or refuse, treatment.

It is not uncommon within general practice for a minor to refuse treatment, for example an immunization, but for the parent to give consent. Legally, if the parents have given consent, the nurse may give the injection, although forcing the child to be immunized against his will could be construed as criminal assault (Kline, 1995). If the child fully understands the implications of the vaccine and has a valid reason for refusing, the nurse should heed the child's request.

Conversely, a child may give consent for a vaccine but the parent refuse. If the child is under 16 years of age, has the maturity to understand the implications and wishes to have the vaccine, the nurse may legally give it (Kline, 1995).

> **Activity 1.3: An unaccompanied 14-year-old boy presents in the surgery with a laceration that could develop tetanus following a football injury. He is due for his school-leaving vaccination. Practice policy is to vaccinate only with consent of the parent or guardian. Consider the legal implications and prepare a protocol for future management of this scenario to discuss at the next practice meeting.**

The subject of consent in minors was raised during the Gillick case of 1981 (Cox, 1994). The issue of prescribing oral contraception to under-age girls without parental consent is a major issue (see Chapter 7). The Gillick case resulted in the court ruling that the main concern was the health of young girls and the need to protect them from the possible harmful effects of sexual intercourse. Parents have duties to their children, but children also have rights. The court ruled that any parental rights were terminated when the child achieved sufficient understanding and intelligence to make an informed decision about medical treatment, hence the term 'Gillick competent'. A child's ability to consent is not based just on age, but also on maturity and understanding.

The key issue in child consent is that a child who is capable of making a reasoned decision has a right to be involved in the de-cision-making process. Children need to be fully informed in the same way as does any other client (Rumbold, 1993).

The nurse's role

Nurses can play a crucial part in helping clients to enjoy more equality with doctors in issues of consent (Box 1.4). The nurse has the ability to explain clinical information clearly and listen to clients' anxieties and concerns. Nurses also have the ability to real-ize that consent is an emotional and rational process (Alderson, 1995). The Code of Professional Conduct (UKCC, 1992a) offers guidelines on consent, although the main goal is to enable members of the profession to exercise accountability and respons-ibility: it does not dictate actions. The Code states that nurses must safeguard the interests of individual patients; the interests of the public and the patient must predominate over those of the practi-tioner and profession. The UKCC further advises that nurses who think that their clients are insufficiently informed should discuss their concerns with the doctor.

Legal standards of consent are based on the concept of what the reasonable doctor decides to tell the patient. A nurse who gives a client more information about the risks than the doctor wishes could be placed in a difficult position (Rumbold, 1993).

Box 1.4: The role of the nurse in issues of consent for nursing care

The nurse should:

- use language that the client can understand
- ensure that the client understands the procedure/treatment
- utilize an interpreter where necessary – defer a procedure unless the event is life threatening (e.g. cardiac arrest)
- remember that children are capable of giving informed consent
- not undertake any procedure for which consent is not informed
- liaise with the key worker or general practitioner when mental illness or incapacity prevents the client giving informed consent

Summary

The professional trend towards negotiated, autonomous nurse–client health care has enabled a move away from the old paternalistic methods, in which health professionals knew 'what was best for the patient' (Fullbrook, 1994). There still remains, however, a view within some pockets of society that responsiblity for health lies with the health care team when the individual becomes a patient (Waterworth and Luker, 1990). Nurses working within general practice are in an ideal situation to familiarize themselves with their practice population and to guide and inform them on any health care issues.

Regardless of any legal duty, the nurse has a moral and professional duty to ensure that clients are competent to make a decision when asked, having considered the overall benefits to the patient.

Key points:

1. A person must be fully informed to be able to consent to a procedure.
2. A person must have the mental capacity in order to be fully informed.
3. Children have a right to be involved in their health care.
4. Treatment without consent may be considered assault.

Respect for patient autonomy in general practice

It is essential that health care workers understand the concept of autonomy in order to individualize health care. Although the terms 'autonomy' and 'self-determination' are often used interchangeably in ethical textbooks, autonomy will be used throughout the following text.

The terms 'client' and 'patient' are both used to refer to persons consulting a doctor or nurse. For convenience, the term 'patient' will be used in this text, although it is recognized that many people seen in general practice are 'well people'.

The reader is directed to Beauchamp and Childress (1989) for an in-depth discussion on ethical theory. This section will consider the general issues of autonomy pertinent to practice nurses.

What is autonomy?

'Autonomy' is derived from the Greek *autos* ('self') and *nomos* ('rule', 'governance' or 'law') (Beauchamp and Childress, 1989, p. 67). An autonomous person has the ability to be able to choose for himself or, more extensively, to be able to formulate and carry out his own plans or policies. The autonomous person also has the ability to govern his conduct by rules and values:

> Dutiful citizens are not expected to comply with authoritative commands without provision of reasons and merely because authorities have spoken. (Beauchamp and Childress, 1989, p. 70).

Respect for client autonomy requires the recognition that an individual has the capacity to determine his own destiny.

Activity 1.4: Reflect on a recent situation in your practice when a patient was not involved in his treatment plan. Consider how this situation could have been managed to enable the individual to exert his autonomy.

Ethical issues

The principle of autonomy is commonly regarded as the first principle of contemporary biomedical ethics. Within health care, autonomy can occur only if the patient has at his disposal the necessary information to consider a course of treatment consistent with his beliefs and wishes. Nurses are also autonomous people who do not blindly follow orders but respect their patients' wishes. Autonomy of the nurse and autonomy of the patient appear to be increasingly interdependent.

The principles of autonomy and individuality would suggest that patients should be entitled to information about their condition. However, English law does not give patients the right to know everything about their treatment.

Although the Access to Health Records Act 1990 extended access of patients to their medical records, this access is permitted only at a practitioner's discretion. Handwritten patient notes are often difficult to read, which reduces the benefits of access to medical records.

Bird and White (1995) suggest that health care professionals must provide all the appropriate information required by a prudent patient to make an informed choice, even when it is not requested. This is contrary to the belief that it is a denial of autonomy to force unwanted information on those who have clearly indicated that they do not want it (Lindley, 1991).

Sharing information with patients

Health care professionals have a moral obligation to give patients as much unbiased information as possible with which to make informed autonomous decisions (Rowson, 1993). It is unfortunate that some professionals consider it morally acceptable to give selected information to a patient, believing it to be in the best interests of the patient to do so. This may deny the individual a chance to make an informed choice, reduce his autonomy and increase anxiety. It may also result in a loss of trust and confidence in the profession.

Refusal to disclose relevant information may deprive people of the power to make important decisions affecting their lives. This leads to dilemma in truth-telling.

Where a doctor fails to answer questions about diagnosis and prognosis truthfully, the nurse is expected to refer these questions back to the practitioner (UKCC, 1992a). She may, however, feel comfortable to field some questions by determining the patient's current knowledge and then answer appropriately. Many nurses will have been asked, 'Have I got cancer?' at some time during their career, and found it difficult to find the right answer.

Although there may be occasions when beneficence overrides respect for autonomy, i.e. acting for the patient's good, there should be few occasions for this to affect nursing care. These issues may become more relevant as the nurse's role in general practice expands.

> **Activity 1.5: Mr White is a 55-year-old manual worker. During a routine health check, you discover that his blood pressure is 170/110 mmHg. He asks you what this means and whether it is serious. Consider what information you want Mr White to share with you and what you are competent and comfortable to share with him. You may achieve increased compliance in lifestyle management if you discuss the implications of unmanaged hypertension. You may, however, increase his anxiety. Justify your decision to share or withhold unbiased information from your patient.**

Competence to consent

Informed consent and autonomy are linked by the presumption that mature adults are expected to be mentally competent and have a capacity for autonomy. There is a moral requirement to show respect for this autonomy.

If the patient has the capacity, it is necessary to ensure that he understands the nature and consequences of a choice. Efforts to dissuade the patient are acceptable, and even morally obligatory in some instances, as long as they are not coercive or manipulative. The nurse has a role in helping family and carers to come to terms with a patient's choice and to respect it.

A concern with patient autonomy as an ethical issue has posed problems in the delivery of care. Wright and Levac (1992) consider that it is arrogant, insulting and violent to label families as non-compliant when they do not respond to nursing intervention.

It is important that the individual is able to make a voluntary decision about his treatment. Consent obtained through coercion or manipulation is not regarded as true consent. A patient refused repeat asthma therapy unless he stops smoking is coerced into a recommended course of action. Manipulation includes giving information to influence the individual, or withholding information that alters a person's understanding. This is then not informed consent. It could be argued that, in some instances, nurses who encourage parents to allow their children to be vaccinated have used an element of (unintentional) manipulation to achieve this result.

> **Activity 1.6: Practice policy is to vaccinate all asthmatic and diabetic patients with pneumococcal vaccine. Consider the ethical implications of this policy. Devise an argument to present to the practice meeting for respecting patients' autonomy. This may require a modification of the initial policy. For example, eligible patients could have an information leaflet and/or discussion about the vaccine's benefits and side effects. The patient could then make an informed decision on whether or not to accept the offer.**

The non-autonomous patient

Some people prefer not to make a decision about their treatment but to rely on the doctor or nurse to make that decision. These people are described as being non-autonomous. Seedhouse (1988) suggests that many people are content to be instructed, although independent choosing should be encouraged. If it is clear that it is the patient's own wish to leave the decision-making to the professional, this decision should be respected. A patient who is very ill may choose to be non-autonomous only until his health improves.

Refusal of treatment

An 'action of battery' is a legal suit that may be brought against a nurse if treatment is given in the face of an explicit refusal to treatment (McHale, 1995). There is no power in statute or case law to remove a patient to hospital for treatment unless he falls under the Mental Health Act 1983. When a patient declines care, the refusal should be respected. Although it is hoped that practice nurses will not encounter this scenario, they must be aware of the implications of such action.

Patient autonomy and the practice nurse

Although lay people are becoming more interested in and know-ledgable about their bodies, their illnesses and possible therapies, far too many people are left in the dark about what is actually wrong with them and possible options for treatment (Snell, 1995).

Health-related topics regularly appear in national and local news-papers, and many weekly and monthly magazines. Some people may feel the need to be more involved in any decisions about their current or proposed care, although it should be remembered that others prefer to be directed by health care professionals.

The Patient's Charter (DoH, 1993) has led to increased patient expectation. A positive step to enhance patient autonomy is to provide patients with information about their illness and treatment.

Essentially, all nursing actions invade a person's privacy, and although most of these actions are considered necessary, and consent is given implicitly, it should not be taken for granted. The patient should exercise the right to say 'No'.

Involving patients in making decisions is said to improve health and promote patient welfare (Chadwick and Tadd, 1992). 'Real care' involves a partnership of nurse and patient or client. Chadwick and Tadd suggest that using the word 'client' instead of 'patient' implies that the person receiving care is an autonomous chooser. It could be argued that a 'client' is a person who is paying for a service. Within health care, private patients pay at the point of use, whilst those receiving NHS treatment pay through their national insurance contributions.

Patients from higher social classes receive more explanations voluntarily than do those from lower social classes, although demand for information and advice is widespread among all social groups (Townsend et al., 1992). The issue of communication may need addressing to ensure that all patients are empowered to be autonomous, whatever their social group, ethnicity or disability. The services of an interpreter may be required to enable an informed decision to be made.

Patients should be offered information which, if accepted, must be delivered at a level the patient and family or carer can understand, with audiovisual or written support for patients to read and absorb at their own pace.

Refusal to consent is an area that may cause concern within general practice. Women who refuse to attend for cervical smears may be harrassed by doctors who strive to reach a specified target level for payment. This practice violates their autonomy and should be discouraged. Nurses have an important role in informing women about cervical screening and supporting those who refuse the test for any reason.

Although the advantages of encouraging patient autonomy are recognized, there are several reasons why nurses may be reluctant to encourage such participation (Box 1.5) (Saunders, 1995).

Box 1.5: Reasons why nurses may be reluctant to encourage patient autonomy

- Feeling threatened by the patient having a stronger role in the partnership
- Being asked too many questions
- Belief that patients should put their trust in the nursing and medical staff
- Fear that the nurse's role will be eroded as more patients self-care
- A view that tasks are completed faster and more thoroughly if the patient remains a passive recipient of care

---

Encouraging autonomy is time consuming, but it can result in improved treatment compliance, which may save further surgery appointments and/or reduce patient morbidity (Edwards, 1996).

Autonomy in health promotion

The need to develop the confidence and competence of lay people to take responsibility for their own health, by state-directed health education and health promotion, was addressed by the World Health Organization's Health for All 2000 strategy, although the whole concept of health education raises ethical questions (Thompson et al., 1994).

Health educators have to respect the rights and autonomy of the individual to choose his lifestyle, despite their primary remit for the prevention of disease. Health promotion features strongly in a general practice workload. Advice on lifestyle changes must be individualized and sensitive, respecting the client's culture and social values. The role of the nurse includes spending time with the patient identifying his social norms and values. A person who makes an informed decision not to adopt a healthy lifestyle following a health screening programme should have his decision respected.

Advocacy and autonomy

Many of the arguments surrounding advocacy and nursing have been addressed by Gates (1994). As an advocate for autonomy, the nurse assists the patient to make an authentic decision that meets his own values and lifestyle. The nurse may also act as the patient's advocate if decisions made by others conflict with the person's wishes. Unfortunately, budgetary restraints may decrease client autonomy in some general practices. If a nurse is unable to act on a patient's behalf, she should refer him to a local independent advocacy scheme. The Community Health Council will have information about local advocates.

Autonomy and trainees

The ethical issues of using patients during nurse or doctor training have been discussed by Thompson et al. (1994). Pre- and post-registration nursing students, medical students and general practitioner trainees receive some of their training in general practice. They develop many skills, including taking cervical smears and carrying out minor surgery. Patients should be allowed to consent to or refuse examination or treatment by a learner, even when this restricts training opportunities, without this decision affecting their future care. This also applies to trainees 'sitting in' on consultations. A patient's permission should be sought prior to the learner meeting the patient.

Living wills

Living wills are achieving recognition as valid documents in civil law. They are advance directives that allow patients to refuse treatment in advance or to state their preference for treatment to continue should they become too ill to make their own choice or to express that choice.

Practice nurses are unlikely to follow advance directives within their professional role but may be asked to read, witness or discuss the concept of the living will during a consultation. For further information, the reader is directed to 'Living Wills: Guidance for Nurses' (RCN, 1994).

One of the central aims of nursing today is the development of autonomous practitioners who are better able to assist patients to cope and take decisions. Individualized patient care recognizes the patient as a person rather than an object of clinical practice.

The patient's role is changing from one of grateful recipient to active consumer. It has been argued that although completely autonomous decision-making is a myth, the person seeking the informed consent should allow the individual the freedom to make his own choice, although deciding a person's autonomous interests is a difficult matter (Cook, 1992).

The Code of Professional Conduct, Section 5, reinforces the nurses' role in respecting patients' involvement in the planning and delivery of care (UKCC, 1992a). Nurses have a duty to inform patients of their rights and assist them to ask questions and express their opinions. Nurses who are not comfortable in this role may benefit from reflection and training to develop the necessary skills to fulfil this duty.

The nurse has a duty to respect patients who prefer to be non-autonomous and passive in their care, i.e. who prefer the nurse or doctor to make all the decisions about their care. Patients should be offered information about their disease, treatment and general management, and be allowed to accept or reject this offer (Figure 1.3).

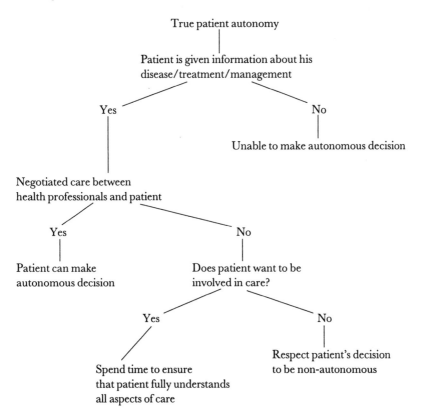

Figure 1.3: True patient autonomy.

The fear of patient litigation may increase patient autonomy in the future.

Respect for the individual requires that each person must be treated as unique and as equal to every other person. There are few areas in which a person cannot, if they choose, be autonomous in their health care.

Key points:

1. Patients have to be informed to be enabled to make a choice.
2. Some patients (non-autonomous patients) prefer not to make a decision, relying on the nurse's judgement.
3. The nurse must respect a decision to refuse care or treatment.
4. The nurse may need to act as an advocate to enable a patient to assert his autonomy.

References

Alderson P (1995) Consent to surgery: the role of the nurse. Nursing Standard 9(8): 38–40.

Beardshaw V (1981) Conscientious Objectors at Work. London: Social Audit.

Beauchamp TL, Childress JF (1989) Principles of Biomedical Ethics, 3rd Edn. Oxford: Oxford University Press.

Bergman R (1981) Accountability: definition and dimensions. International Nursing Review 28(2): 53–9.

Bird A, White J (1995) Consent and the adult patient. An ethical perspective – patient autonomy. In Tingle J, Cribb A (Eds) Nursing Law and Ethics. Oxford: Blackwell Science.

Black D (1990) Confidentiality of Personal Health Information. Report of an Interprofessional Working Group. London: BMA.

Burnard P, Chapman CM (1988) Professional and Ethical Issues in Nursing. Chichester: John Wiley & Sons.

Carlisle D (1992) Scope for extensions. Nursing Times 88(37): 26–9.

Castledine G (1992) New Code of Professional Conduct: how it affects you. British Journal of Nursing 1(6): 296–300.

Chadwick R, Tadd W (1992) Ethics and Nursing Practice. London: Macmillan.

Chambers Dictionary (1993) Edinburgh: Chambers Publishers Ltd.

Cook T (1992) The nurse and informed consent. Senior Nurse 12(2): 41–5.

Cox D (1994) Ethics and the law. GP (September): 44–6.

Department of Health (1993) The Patient's Charter. London: HMSO.

Department of Health (1994) The Heathrow Debate 1993: The Challenges for Nursing and Midwifery in the 21st Century. London: HMSO.

Edwards M (1996) Drug compliance: a continuing problem. Practice Nursing 7(20): 21–2.

Evans A (1993) Accountability: a core concept for primary nursing. Journal of Clinical Nursing 2: 231–4.

Fullbrook P (1994) Assessing mental competence of patients and relatives. Journal of Advanced Nursing 20: 457–61.

Gates B (1994) Advocacy. A Nurse's Guide. London: Scutari Press.

Hanford L (1993) Ethics and disability. British Journal of Nursing 2(19): 979–82.

Hepworth S (1989) Professional judgement and nurse education. Nurse Education Today 9: 408–12.

Jones M (1996) Accountability in Practice: A Guide to Professional Responsibility for Nurses in General Practice. Salisbury: Quay Books.

Jones S (1994) Ethics in Midwifery. London: CV Mosby.

Kline R (1995) Immunisation: at the sharp end. Health Visitor 68(10): 412.

Korgaonkar G, Tribe D (1994) Confidentiality, patients and the law. British Journal of Nursing 3(2): 91–3.

Lindley R (1991) Informed consent and the ghost of Bolam. In Brazier M, Lobjoit M (Eds) Protecting the Vulnerable. Autonomy and Consent in Health Care. London: Routledge.

McHale J (1995) Consent and the adult patient. The legal perspective. In Tingle J, Cribb A (Eds) Nursing Law and Ethics. Oxford: Blackwell Science.

Milburn A (1997) The health of the nation. An interview with Alan Milburn, Minister of State for Health. MSF at work (Autumn/Winter).

National Health Service Management Executive (1990) A Guide to Consent for Examination or Treatment. London: NHMSE.

Orme L, Maggs C (1993) Decision-making in clinical practice: how do expert nurses, midwives and health visitors make decisions? Nurse Education Today 13: 270–6.

Pyne R (1988) On being accountable. Health Visitor 61: 173–5.

Pyne R (1992) Accountability in principle and in practice. British Journal of Nursing 1(6): 304.

Pyne R (1994) Empowerment through use of the Code of Professional Conduct. British Journal of Nursing 3(12): 631–4.

Rowson R (1993) Informed consent. In Tschudin V (Ed.) Ethics, Nurses and Patients. London: Scutari Press.

Royal College of Nursing (1992) The Value of Nursing. London: RCN.

Royal College of Nursing (1994) Living Wills: Guidance for Nurses. London: RCN.

Rumbold G (1993) Ethics in Nursing Practice. London: Baillière Tindall.

Saunders P (1995) Encouraging patients to take part in their own care. Nursing Times 91(5): 42–3.

Seedhouse D (1988) Ethics: The Heart of Health Care. Chichester: John Wiley & Sons.

Snell J (1995) Keeping your patients informed. Nursing Times 9(43): 40–2.

Tadd GV (1991) Where are the whistleblowers? Nursing Times 87(1): 42–4.

Tadd V (1994) Professional codes: an exercise in tokenism? Nursing Ethics 1(1): 15–23.

Thiroux J (1980) Ethics, Theory and Practice, 2nd Edn. Encino, CA: Glencoe Publishing.

Thompson IA, Melia KM, Boyd KM (1994) Nursing Ethics, 3rd Edn. London: Churchill Livingstone.

Townsend P, Davidson N, Whitehead M (1992) Inequalities in Health. London: Penguin Books.

Tschudin V (1994a) Nursing ethics 4: Theories and principles. Nursing Standard 9(2): 52–5.

Tschudin V (1994b) Nursing ethics 6: Particular features. Nursing Standard 9(4): 52–5.

United Kingdom Central Council for Nursing, Midwifery and Health Visiting (1987) Confidentiality: A UKCC Advisory Paper. London: UKCC.

United Kingdom Central Council for Nursing, Midwifery and Health Visiting (1989) Exercising Accountability: A UKCC Advisory Document. London: UKCC.

United Kingdom Central Council for Nursing, Midwifery and Health Visiting (1992a) Code of Professional Conduct for the Nurse, Midwife and Health Visitor, 3rd Edn. London: UKCC.

United Kingdom Central Council for Nursing, Midwifery and Health Visiting (1992b) The Scope of Professional Practice. London: UKCC.

United Kingdom Central Council for Nursing, Midwifery and Health Visiting (1996) Guidelines for Professional Practice. London: UKCC.

Waterworth S, Luker K (1990) Reluctant collaborators. Do patients want to be involved in decisions concerning care? Journal of Advanced Nursing 15: 971–6.

Wright LM, Levac AMC (1992) The non-existence of non-compliant families: the influence of Humberto Maturana. Journal of Advanced Nursing 17(8): 913–17.

Young AP (1989) Legal Problems in Nursing Practice. London: Chapman & Hall.

Further reading

Beauchamp TL, Childress JF (1989) Principles of Biomedical Ethics, 3rd Edn. Oxford: Oxford University Press.

British Medical Association (1993) Medical Ethics Today: Its Practice and Philosophy. London: BMA.

Chadwick R, Tadd W (1992) Ethics and Nursing Practice. London: Macmillan.

Downie RS, Calman KC (1994) Health Respect. Ethics in Health Care, 2nd Edn. Oxford: Oxford University Press.

Faulker C (1985) Whose Body Is It? The Troubling Issue of Informed Consent. London: Virago.

Harris J (1985) The Value of Life: An Introduction to Medical Ethics. London: Routledge.

Jones M (1996) Accountability in Practice: A Guide to Professional Responsibility for Nurses in General Practice. Salisbury: Quay Books.

Seedhouse D (1988) Ethics: The Heart of Health Care. Chichester: John Wiley & Sons.

Tschudin V (1992) Ethics in Nursing, 2nd Edn. Oxford: Butterworth-Heinemann.

Chapter 2
Management

Pat Tweed and Marilyn Edwards

An understanding of the culture and structure of organizations offers an insight into some of the difficulties the reader may encounter within the workplace. Although this may appear to be a complex subject, each aspect is broken down into comprehensible sections to which the reader can relate. It is hoped that this chapter may encourage each nurse to look objectively at his/her employing organization and be involved in a team/practice management plan.

The effective management of an organization includes time management and quality issues. This chapter examines time management in general practice, and although the emphasis is on the role of the practice nurse, it has repercussions for all the staff.

Quality means meeting the needs of the people in the system. Audit can provide the evidence of efficient and effective quality health care practice that meets the goals and objectives of the organization.

Organizations

'Organisations are social arrangements for the controlled performance of collective goals' (Buchanan and Huczynski, 1985), but these are usually the reconciled aspirations of individuals rather than of the organization as a body.

All organizations have a structure, even if none is apparent. Drucker (1974) tells us that 'structure is a means for obtaining the objectives and goals of an organisation'. This section will look at different cultures that exist in organizations and the way in which these are reflected in the management structures of general practice, where internal and external factors have combined to influence that structure in recent years.

Consideration of current organizational structures may enable the reader to recognize the prevailing culture of his or her organization and how to work more effectively within it, seek to change it or even to recognize the incompatibility of personal beliefs and those of an employer.

Handy (1993) suggests that cultures stem from deeply held beliefs about the organization of work, the exercise of authority and how people should be rewarded and controlled. Cultures are founded and built by the dominant groups in an organization, and their appropriateness will change as the people within the groups and their relative power changes. This can be seen in many general practices where the combination of the organizational changes in the NHS, increased patient expectation and the vast expansion of screening and preventive health services have overturned the existing culture, and the former management structure has not been adequately replaced.

Technology

The technology of an organization greatly influences its structure. General practice is a combination of routine and non-routine work, the former, according to Handy (1993), being more generally suited to a role culture and the latter to a power or task culture. Routine, programmable operations such as screening and immunization are most effectively carried out within a hierarchical structure, in which the work is controlled by policies and protocols, and the areas of discretion are narrow.

However, the individualized care needed for the encouragement of lifestyle change or for dealing with chronic disease is more suited to a matrix structure based on teams that incorporate nurses, doctors and other health and social care professionals, with a variety of expertise.

General practice also requires the ability to deal with rapidly changing and emergency situations in which there is no time to wait for instructions or to discuss the problem with team colleagues. Decisions must be made and action taken independently by confident and competent individuals, who are more likely to be found within a power culture where they are used to being 'trusted to get on with the job' (Handy, 1993).

The vastly differing range of technologies and personality types in a small organization such as general practice may be a significant deterrent to the formulation of a common management structure.

Authority, leadership and autonomy

Authority is related to status and implies 'a right to control and judge the action of others, whilst leadership is the exercise of the power conferred by that right' (Torrington and Weightman, 1989).

A leader may inspire through the shaping and sharing of a vision, described by Macgregor Burns (1978) as 'transformational leadership', or results may be achieved through allowing the follower to know what is expected and trusting him to achieve it. Autonomy is that freedom of action which subordinates see as being necessary to be effective in their roles.

Status

Status in a general practice may stem from a title, either bestowed by a professional organization or the work organization, such as 'doctor', 'sister' or 'practice manager'; being granted from knowledge or ability, such as the recognition of special knowledge of a particular condition, so that others seek advice from that person; or arising from financial control attached to the post of fund manager.

Organizational cultures

Handy (1993) identified four main types of organizational culture (Box 2.1).

Box 2.1: Organizational cultures and structures (Handy, 1993)

Culture	Structure
power	web
role	Greek temple
task	matrix (net)
person	cluster

The power and task cultures are closely related to those described by Schein (1986), in his conceptual studies of organizations, as organization A, in which 'ideas come from individuals and people are considered responsible, motivated and capable of governing themselves'.

The role culture equates with Schein's organization B, in which 'truth comes from older, wiser and higher-status members', and staff 'loyally carry out directions'.

The person culture usually has no identifiable organizational structure but is often seen as a cluster of individuals.

Power culture

This culture is usually found in small, entrepreneurial organizations where the structure is a web with a central power source (Figure 2.1), usually derived from the personality of the leader. This could be the senior partner in a general medical practice.

Rays of power and influence radiate from the centre, connected by functional or specialist strings (nursing, administration and fund-holding), each co-ordinated by a key individual. Effectiveness depends on the person in the centre and the selection of power-orientated, politically minded risk-takers in the functional strings who are allowed to get on with the job.

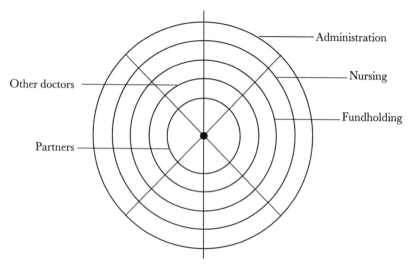

Figure 2.1: Power culture – the web (adapted from Handy, 1993).

These cultures judge by results and are tolerant of means; there are few rules or procedures and little bureaucracy. Lines of communication are often informal and run between the centre and the co-ordinators. The atmosphere is competitive, and progress for the individual is through 'horizontal tracking' (Handy, 1991).

More of the same or different work at the same level allows for the development of wider expertise as there are few opportunities for vertical promotion in such a structure.

This type of structure can be found in some general practices, but many of the people who have worked in public services such as health find this type of structure demoralizing and difficult to understand, either due to its lack of formal rules, hierarchies and systems of communication, or because of a psychological attachment to the underlying culture and a lack of understanding of management.

The central person needs to choose people who think in the same way as himself in order to ensure that the objectives of the organization, or the centre's personal objectives, will be achieved with the minimum of bureaucracy or need for central control over processes.

Such organizations have the ability to move quickly when threatened, which, in the current climate of discontinuous change (Handy, 1991), can enable them to take advantage of immediate opportunities, but this will happen only if there is strong central leadership.

In a web structure, the vision will not be realized without the right choice of key individuals in the specialist strings.

Role culture

The role culture, with its representative structure of a Greek temple (Figure 2.2), is dependent on the strength of its pillars; in health service organizations, these might be finance, administration, medicine and nursing.

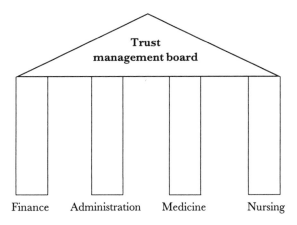

Figure 2.2: Role culture – the temple (adapted from Handy, 1993).

The pillars are co-ordinated at the top by a narrow band of senior management, and the work of the pillars is controlled by rules and procedures that, if followed, will ensure the result. 'The job description or role is often more important than the person who fulfils it' (Handy, 1993). This perception does little to encourage extra effort or innovation; indeed, these are often actively discouraged. Influence comes from the position held rather than from expertise or personality.

Communication is clear and vertical, usually top-down, with lots of paperwork. Although the system tends to be slow and unwieldy, it provides security and visible advancement up the ladder.

Role culture is common in the hospital services, particularly since the introduction of general management. It is not common in general practice, largely because of the small size and absence of rules and established procedures, but this may change (Berger and Rosner, 1996).

The growing enthusiasm for managed care programmes that promote only evidence-based treatments would be most easily applied in such a structure. Doctors and nurses would work to defined protocols and procedures; task-orientated, providing only proven cost-effective treatment, with little respect for the value of experience and professional skill.

Task culture

The task culture seeks to bring together the appropriate people and resources to do the job, and, with its emphasis on results, teamwork and the devolution of power, is most in tune with current ideologies, a view supported by Handy (1993).

Influence is expert rather than personal or positional. It is also more widely distributed, so that each member of the team feels more empowered. Teams, task forces and project groups are formed for a purpose and disbanded or reformed when the task is complete. The accompanying structure is a matrix or net (Figure 2.3), the power and influence lying at the 'knots' of the net, where the relevant resources and expertise meet.

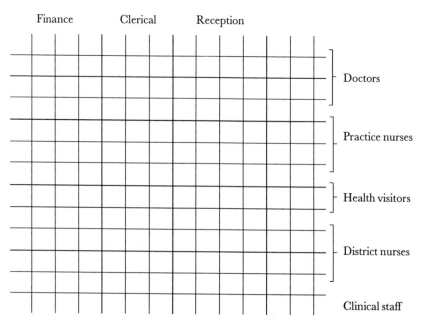

Figure 2.3: Task culture – the matrix (adapted from Handy, 1993). Appropriate staff with necessary levels of authority come together as a team to complete a task.

Communication is horizontal and vertical, and may be problematic if different directorates or professional groups have differing philosophies or internal structures. Authority is devolved to the grass roots, with fewer procedures and a flattened hierarchy.

The current move toward a primary care-based NHS, which is likely to continue whatever the prevailing political mood, highlights the contribution to be made to health care by non-medical members of the primary health care team.

This may be through practice-based contracts (NHSE, 1996) and single budgets, allowing practices to manage all their resources to purchase health and social care. Task culture would give the necessary flexibility to develop teamworking and provide a more exciting and fulfilling career path for primary care nurses.

This flexibility could permit a group to be formed in a practice to develop a strategy for the prevention of coronary heart disease; this may need to change its membership when it moves to set standards for the control of hyperlipidaemia, for which different expertise is needed.

Person culture

The individual is the central point within the person culture. The structure, if one exists, serves only to assist the individuals within it.

Handy (1993) defines the psychological contract by stating that 'the organisation is subordinate to the individual and depends on the individual for its existence'. If such individuals decide to band together for the furtherance of a mutual interest, the structure (the group practice) would resemble a loose cluster. This culture has existed in professional practices of architects, solicitors and, more recently, general medical practice.

Single-handed doctors have come together to form partnerships of independent contractors providing an individualistic service to a group of patients, supported by 'ancillary staff', which include nurses. This is the preferred culture of many general practitioners. The power base is expert, and individuals 'do what they are good at', a situation described by Strong and Robinson (1990) as 'rampant individualism'. Authority is generally seen as being related to superior status – in this case that of the professional, the doctor.

Hospital consultants have also preferred this culture, feeling little allegiance to the organization, but instead to their patients, with few means available to control their performance (Handy, 1993).

The change in political climate has forced change upon both these groups, and they are now obliged to operate in a different type of organization. This has provided nursing with the opportunity to ensure that its contribution is recognized by doctors and other primary care professionals (DoH, 1994).

> **Activity 2.1: Identify the culture reflected in the structure of your organization. Which type of technology does your practice deal with best: is it the routine programmable work, the individual teamwork or the emergency, crisis interventions? Does your assessment of the culture appear to fit? Now consider a hypothetical general practice and how recent changes in health service policy, affecting the culture and structure of the organization, present opportunities for nurses to become equal partners in primary care provision.**

The Riverside practice

To study these principles further, let us take the example of the hypothetical Riverside practice.

History and ownership

Since the inception of the NHS in 1948, GPs have been self-employed, independent contractors to the family health services authority and its predecessors, and now directly to the district health authority, providing primary medical services. Unlike other health care providers, the medical partners often own the premises and employ all the staff.

Registered nurses have been employed by the Riverside practice for nearly 20 years. The contribution that practice nurses have made to patient care was largely unrecognized until the establishment of the new general practitioner contract in 1990. Practice nurses had always been classed as ancillary staff, alongside clerical and administrative personnel, thus denying their professional status.

External influences

During the 1980s, several government White Papers emphasized the importance of primary health care teams, 'Promoting Better Health' (DoH, 1987) being the most important in relation to general practice.

The development of health promotion clinics at the end of the 1980s, and the targets set by the aforementioned new general practitioner contract, gave a new importance to the employment of practice nurses, and numbers doubled. However, the culture of the Riverside practice remained unchanged, the nurses being used only to earn money for the partners, who continued to work independently, sometimes even of each other.

General practitioner fundholding, introduced to the Riverside practice in 1992 as a result of the White Paper 'Working for Patients' (DoH, 1989), increased the power of the general practitioners. All fundholding practices had to submit business plans, and contracts were placed based on historical practice data owing to a lack of information on true need. At the Riverside practice, only the fund manager and the partners contributed to the plans or the contracts, and there was no discussion amongst other team members of the success or otherwise of the operation.

Communication

No formal channels of communication existed at the practice until 1993, a situation common to the person culture (Handy, 1993). Discussions of patient care or operational problems took place on an *ad hoc* basis over coffee and were frequently interrupted. The office manager held a tight grip on all information relating to reception and clerical work, thereby denying the staff any power to influence practice. The fourth tier of Maslow's pyramid of need (Maslow, 1943) is 'esteem', based on capability and respect from others; this was not evident at the practice.

Activity 2.2: Consider how communication channels could be improved in your practice.

Structure of the organization

Since the Riverside practice was still clearly a person culture without stated objectives or goals, the absence of a definable structure continued. Attempts to create a matrix structure to devolve responsibility to different sections of the workforce failed.

The unwillingness to give away power to the teams, and a lack of interest on the part of the partners, prevented any change from taking place. Handy (1993) states that 'control mechanisms or even management hierarchies are impossible in person cultures, except by mutual consent', and such mutuality was clearly absent.

Authority and leadership

Torrington and Weightman (1989) suggest that, being related to superior status, authority implies a right to control and judge the actions of others. The staff at the Riverside practice recognized the authority of the partners but did not feel able to rely on them for support and guidance with problems in the work situation.

The partners may have felt that their authority demanded 'deference to them as superior kinds of people', a view that the staff rejected, thereby rejecting the doctors' right to control or judge the actions of other staff.

In 1992, Dr Jones drew up a practice 'mission statement' that was not shared with the rest of the practice. This conflicted with Macgregor Burns' (1978) assertion that 'the vision needs to be shared, not imposed by the central powerhead' and that 'it must be related to their work, not to some grand design in which they feel no part'.

There was no clear evidence of leadership within the practice when considered against the eight main elements of effective leadership identified by Adair (1988a) (Box 2.2). A succession of developments were brought about by the personal influence of one partner who had taken control and changed the culture to one of personal power, without a supporting structure apart from a financial management system essential for fundholding status.

Box 2.2: The key elements of the functional approach to effective leadership (Adair, 1988a)

- defining the task
- planning
- briefing
- controlling
- evaluating
- motivating
- organizing
- setting an example

Status

Power resulting from expertise and knowledge may be very narrow and not available in other areas of work so that the expert in one area has no control over other aspects of his job. The nurses' expertise in family planning and asthma care was acknowledged by the partners, but the nursing contribution was rejected in other areas, such as planning for prevention of coronary heart disease.

Goals and objectives

Buchanan and Huczynski (1985) hold that 'organisations do not have goals, only people have goals'. This theory would certainly fit the climate at Riverside, where the lead partner had many diverse plans for the future of the practice that were not shared with or supported by the other partners, who still saw themselves as experts 'doing what they were good at' rather than as leaders or managers.

Activity 2.3: Does your practice have a shared philosophy of care? Are you aware of any written aims and objectives of practice? Do you know what they are, or can you find out?

The environment

The community nurses and health visitors at Riverside, although practice based, were still managed by a trust, 'their day to day work activity still driven by trust requirements and information systems' (Rix and Elwyn, 1996).

At least one trust, and others now following (Cohen, 1996), has marketed the services of community health professionals to general practices, through contracts that transfer day-to-day management to the practice. A team leader is appointed within the practice, but the trust retains responsibility for professional support, education and training.

The future

The person culture and unstructured management system at the Riverside practice cannot produce the outcomes required by the government from the primary health care services, in terms of either information, uniformity of treatment or prevention of disease (NHSE, 1996). The political and financial pressure necessitates a change to a different culture and structure that can deliver the outcomes.

The dynamic nature of current change rules out the role culture and its hierarchical structure, which requires stability and defined patterns of work. A power culture and its web structure, with the appropriate choice of people in the strings, could be successful, although it may be difficult to find enough of these people in the health care field as ambitious risk-takers do not predominate in the caring professions.

The task culture, expressed as a matrix or net, is probably the most appropriate and would allow for the inclusion of the other health and social care workers within the primary health care team. A web would become too large for efficient management.

Summary

Handy (1993) states that cultures are built by the dominant groups in an organization. As the skill and knowledge of nurses in primary care increases through education and experience, and nurse practitioners, educated to Master's level, take their place alongside their colleagues, the dominance of medical opinion will be tempered by a broader view of health care.

Traditional roles of dominance and deference are being replaced by a more collaborative co-practitioner relationship (Lawley, 1997). The status of the medical practitioner will no longer be seen as superior, as nurses achieve equality of education; then the right to control and judge the work of others will have no justification.

'Task orientation' is a much-maligned term in nursing. It has traditionally been used to describe a philosophy concentrating not on the needs of individuals but on the performance of a nursing procedure. A task culture, on the other hand, concentrates on the needs of individuals or groups and brings together a team of people with the expertise to fulfil those needs. The establishment of a structure that allows this to happen requires the acceptance of a shared philosophy of care, and leadership willing to devolve power to the teams.

Communication can be difficult in a matrix structure, but shared aims and a willingness to give away power, through the sharing of information, should enable a system of communication to be established that will address the needs of team members and produce an effective outcome for the client.

The importance of a culture and structure that promotes the growth of professional teams, with common aims, is supported by 'New World, New Opportunities' (NHSME, 1993), which devotes a whole section to 'teamworking'. It identifies the need for a shared philosophy, the prioritizing of aims and health targets, and the development of a team/practice management plan. Review of outcomes measured against objectives, through the medium of regular meetings, is highlighted as an essential key to progress.

Key points:

1. Organizations must have shared goals and objectives.
2. Communication is the key to good organization.

Quality in primary health care

Quality has been highlighted as a key factor in the future of primary health care (Dorrell, 1996) but it should be an integral part of all health care interventions. There are many papers relating to quality in the hospital setting but limited literature relating to quality in general practice. It is time for practice nurses to redress this imbalance and share their experiences of quality primary health care.

Duty of care

Nurses have a legal and professional duty to care for patients (UKCC, 1996). Despite the increasingly limited resources at the disposal of health service workers, every practitioner has a responsibility for ensuring that patients receive a high level of quality care.

Quality assurance

The purpose of quality assurance is to ensure the consumer of nursing receives a specified degree of excellence through continuous measurement and evaluation (Schmadl, quoted in Sale, 1996, p. 13).

Quality assurance measures the actual level of service provided and is a means of offering an effective, efficient cost-effective service. This includes efforts to modify the provision of these services where appropriate. For example, an audit of patient waiting times may suggest a modification of the surgery appointment system. Many examples of quality assurance tools can be found in textbooks; the reader is directed to the further reading list for an in-depth analysis of the topic. A simple example of quality assurance is shown in Figure 2.4 and expanded further throughout the text.

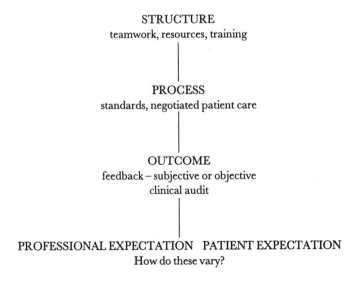

STRUCTURE
teamwork, resources, training

PROCESS
standards, negotiated patient care

OUTCOME
feedback – subjective or objective
clinical audit

PROFESSIONAL EXPECTATION   PATIENT EXPECTATION
How do these vary?

Figure 2.4: Simplified example of quality assurance.

Measuring quality

The six measurable areas that can be addressed to ensure quality in health care (Ranade, 1994) are described below and related to general practice:

1. *Appropriateness*: the service or procedure is one which the individual or population actually needs. A practice profile should highlight the needs of the population (see Chapter 4).
2. *Equity*: services are fairly shared amongst the population who need them. There is documented evidence of inequality in health care between social groups (Townsend et al., 1992).
3. *Accessibility*: services are readily accessible and not compromised by distance or time restraints. Surgeries that operate from 9 am until 5 pm are not accessible for commuters or manual workers, who often work long hours.
4. *Effectiveness*: the services achieve the intended benefit for the individual and for the population. This can be assessed through clinical audit.
5. *Acceptability*: the service satisfies the reasonable expectations of patients, providers and the community. Satisfaction may be viewed subjectively as individuals' expectations can vary according to race, social group and education.
6. *Efficiency*: resources are not wasted on one service or patient to the detriment of another. Self-care, for example in wound management, is an efficient use of resources for some patients in some instances.

Activity 2.4: Choose one area of patient care, for example the prevention of coronary heart disease, and consider whether it meets the six criteria described above. This may help you identify areas for future standard-setting and clinical audit.

Donabedian (1988) suggests that scientific measurement be used where possible, supplementing quantitative measures with qualitative data. His work relates to the theory of structure, process and outcome, which can be applied to many areas of health care (see Figure 2.4).

'Structure' encompasses material and human resources, and includes the environment, supplies and all levels of staff. It can also include methods of peer review and methods of reimbursement.

'Process' denotes what is actually done in giving and receiving care, including the patient's activities in seeking care as well as the practitioner's activities in making a diagnosis.

'Outcome' denotes the effects of care on the patient. Outcome measures reflect total care received, are readily understood and can be used to indicate not just quality of care, but also needs for further or compensatory care. Specified outcomes provide the feedback for future care.

Attree (1993) has explored the concept of quality and offers a framework for quality care that includes Donabedian's principles (Tables 2.1–2.3).

Table 2.1: Structural criteria of quality nursing care

Criteria	Examples
Organizational variables	Concept of care/philosophy of nursing Manpower: numbers, grades, competence, level of education and professional development Accountability, leadership and supervision Patient care episodes, i.e. how often a patient attends for nursing care Resources: human – care, educate; material – equipment, facilities
Patient environment	Physical: buildings and equipment: type, main-tenance and repair, facilities, hygiene Social: atmosphere
Service attributes	Accessibility, equity, acceptability Relevance to need Effectiveness, efficiency and economy

Table 2.2: Process criteria of quality nursing care

Criteria type	Examples
Care functions/processes	Assessment, planning, intervention, recording, evaluation
Interpersonal processes	Effective communication Involvement of patient and family/carer Provision of a supportive environment
Method of organizing work	Accountability, effective co-ordination Individualized, holistic approach to care Nurse/patient-negotiated decision-making

(contd)

Table 2.2: (contd)

Criteria type	Examples
Nurses' professional perspective	Approach to and philosophy of nursing Attitudes, beliefs and values Inclination and time to listen, talk and educate
Nurses' professional practice	Knowledgeable, proficient, clinically and technically competent
Nurses' personal characteristics	Qualities include caring, compassion, concern and respect for patient autonomy

Table 2.3: Outcome criteria of quality nursing care

Criteria type	Examples
Health/wellness level	Morbidity/mortality Improvement/maintenance of health
Functional ability	Physiological, psychological, social
Patient satisfaction	Access, availability, complaints, compliments
Cost-effectiveness/efficiency	Compliance, patient return rate Quality of life
Undesirable events	Accidents and incidents: falls Iatrogenic diseases Infection
Undesirable processes	Medication and recording errors Un-coordinated services

Tables 2.1–2.3 are adapted from Attree (1993) with kind permission from Elsevier Science Ltd, The Boulevard, Langford Lane, Kidlington OX5 1GB, UK.

Standards and criteria

Standards are agreed statements of acceptable, observable, achievable and measurable levels of performance. They may also be called policy statements that specify aims. In health care, they relate to the quality of care relevant to the needs of the population and health care staff. Standards may be set nationally (for example, cervical screening targets), as a district policy (such as an infection control policy relevant to the health of a specific population) or locally (specific to a general practice).

Grol (1993) has developed guidelines for quality in general practice. Although aimed at doctors, the guidelines are relevant to the nurses who may be delegated the task of assuring quality in one form or another. Grol emphasizes the need for teamwork, planning, consensus and scientific validity when developing guidelines.

Criteria are the descriptive statements, or steps, of how the standard will be met and must be specific, clear, achievable and clinically sound (Box 2.3). Although most standards are related to actual health care, there must also be standards or policy statements on all aspects of general practice management. The practice charter may encompass patient expectations other than health.

Box 2.3: Example of standard and criteria in general practice

Standard:
90% of patients receiving thyroxine will be reviewed and have their blood levels assessed at least annually.

Rationale:
To ensure that patients receive therapeutic levels of medication.

Criteria:
• Identify all patients receiving thyroxine – from repeat medication or via disease register
• Check date of last blood test for thyroid stimulating hormone (TSH)
• If not recorded in past 12 months, recall for blood test
• Assess compliance with current medication
• Determine whether or not the patient is symptomatic
• Ensure that the patient is aware of the process for receiving blood results, and advise of annual recall
• Annual recall implemented through manual or computer system

---

Although it is preferable to state that *all* patients should be reviewed annually, a more realistic standard has been set. This can be reviewed following an audit.

Activity 2.5: Consider the standard and criteria in Box 2.3 and modify it to meet the needs of your practice for one aspect of chronic disease management.

Audit

The purpose of audit is to improve the quality of care. Intended performance is compared against actual performance (Figure 2.5), which requires information about the structure, process and outcomes of the area being audited.

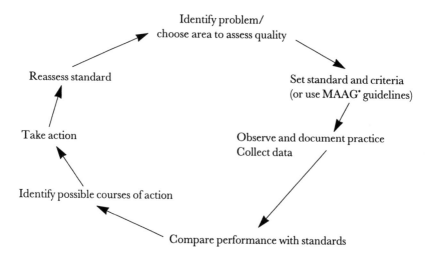

Figure 2.5: An audit cycle. *MAAG (medical audit advisory group) is contactable through the health authority.

A review of the quality system and strategy will highlight whether or not the standards have been achieved, and modifications of priorities, targets and training needs can be proposed and implemented (Ellis and Whittington, 1993).

The chief source of information for measuring quality outcome is the medical records, which should be fully completed and contemporaneous. Recorded data, written or recorded on a computer, can be readily accessed for audit purposes. Audit will identify areas of action for improvement. In the example in Box 2.3, a policy can be implemented to ensure that all patients who require thyroxine therapy receive a therapeutic dose.

The audit may highlight excellent practice, which will motivate the staff to continue a high level of quality care. A deficiency highlighted from an audit should not be viewed negatively but as a positive outcome. This may result in continuing education for medical and nursing staff, and improved effectiveness within the practice team.

Audit need not be a complicated exercise. For example, the quality of minor surgery in general practice may be assessed through documenting the level of post-surgical wound infection (Edwards, 1996). No audit will benefit patient care, or staff development, if staff are not committed to implement recommended changes.

Activity 2.6: Using the model in Figure 2.5 above, identify an area of care within your practice to develop a quality service.

Patient and staff satisfaction

Customers are said to judge quality by comparing the service they receive against expectations of what they should receive, although their views may be subjective (Ranade, 1994). Patient satisfaction may be considered a desirable outcome of care, but a personality clash between patient and health professional may adversely affect this outcome.

Sale (1996) suggests measuring quality of care retrospectively by inviting the patient to discuss his experiences in a post-care interview, which may be structured, unstructured or semi-structured. Although time consuming, patient feedback is necessary for a quality assessment process. As perceptions alter over time, assessing and monitoring quality in health care requires continuous interaction and feedback from patients and staff at all stages of planning and delivering care.

Concurrent measurement (measurement while the patient is in the nurse's care) is more difficult in general practice as the patient is often seen only occasionally. One area that can be observed and modified is patient waiting times.

The needs of staff should not be overlooked. Job satisfaction will affect their contribution to the running of the practice and general patient care, from patients' reception to their exit from the premises. The principles will also apply to staff undertaking home visits.

Quality can be measured through patient satisfaction surveys, documentation, observation and interviewing of staff and patients. Only one method should be chosen to obtain a baseline picture for a procedure. Guidance for undertaking surveys can usually be obtained from the primary health care advisers or institutes of higher education.

Training

Objective measurements highlight excellent practice that may motivate staff, or poor results that can indicate training needs, but if confidential this should not demotivate staff. The results might suggest that the whole team requires some level of training. For example, a high level of inadequate cervical smears indicates the need for further training for relevant staff. Nurses should not undertake tasks in which they have not been appropriately trained and their competencies assessed; training alone does not ensure competence. Peer review requires sensitive handling but should be seen as beneficial to both the practitioner and the patient.

Communication

A clear and well-defined shared vision is essential if people are to work well together (Peters, 1995). An efficient communication channel will enhance the smooth running of a multidisciplinary general practice team. Feedback is essential to determine the expectation and needs of staff and patients or clients.

Practice meetings and in-house training may present opportunities for feedback, discussion and action on complaints, for which practices should have a publicized complaints procedure. Positive feedback will motivate staff to continue their quality improvement.

Reflective practice

The association between thinking and reflection has been recognized (Luft, 1994, p. 178). Many nurses focus on continued action but devote little time to reflecting on this action. Reflection is essential if innovation in nursing practice is to replace traditional methods of care.

Continuing professional development, through either directed or self-directed study, should sow the seeds for reflection. The issues raised throughout this book are intended to encourage the reader to reflect on his or her current practice using simple and useful learning exercises. Outcomes that may initially highlight a negative experience should be viewed as a positive learning experience.

> **Activity 2.7: For one week, keep a note of any areas of patient care, or interpersonal interaction, on which you can reflect. What was particularly good, and what could have been done better? All the experiences should have a positive outcome.**

Summary

The main purpose of quality assurance activity is to improve or maintain the quality of patient care. This involves all members of the practice team, including domestic, clerical and health care staff. Communication is essential to allow areas of concern to be discussed and possible courses of action debated. These discussions should be constructive and non-threatening.

Standards must be agreed following team discussions, using scientific evidence to support decisions. The standards should also be reviewed and updated.

Audit is a useful tool in assessing current practice. It is not a data collection exercise but must be used to improve patient care. Writing standards and undertaking audit are time-consuming processes but are integral to nurses' professional development.

Reflective practice is a positive way in which nurses can promote quality health care. It must be recognized that patients' expectations may differ from those of the health carers, and that one person's perception of quality will vary from another's.

Total quality management can be achieved by meeting client needs and achieving continuous improvement. Quality assurance must be synonymous with quality improvement (Peters, 1995).

Key points:

1. The primary objective of quality assurance activity is to improve patient care.
2. Good communication channels, including interpersonal skills, result in the smooth operation of the primary health care team.
3. Training of all staff is essential to develop and maintain skills.
4. Reflective practice is an essential part of professional development in providing quality health care.

Time management

Health care is a diverse and flexible 'business' that does not slot into commercial time management specifications. Time is a precious resource that is irreplaceable and irreversible (Adair, 1988b), and is a key resource necessary for efficient management (Box 2.4). Improved time management may increase efficiency and effectiveness, increase one's feeling of well-being and subsequently reduce stress. Perry and Rowe (1993) report that nurses often fail to achieve time management skills. The reader is offered the opportunity to reflect on his or her own time management skills, which may result in a more efficient working practice rather than increased effort.

Methods and time are closely linked and are related to money. Parkinson's first law and the Pareto principle (Box 2.5) underpin the whole issue of time management and are frequently quoted in management books.

Box 2.4: Resources at the disposal of management

- Manpower
- Money to pay for manpower and materials
- Time
- Materials
- Methods

Box 2.5: Two key definitions in time management

Parkinson's first law
Work expands to fill the time available for the completion of the task

The Pareto Principle
20% of time determines 80% of production – i.e. 20% of effort produces 80% of results

---

The workload of general practice staff is dynamic, changing to meet the demands of regular Department of Health reviews. Is time really a shortage, and inevitable, or could we make better use of the time available with good planning? Pritchard et al. (1986) refer to Parkinson's law, suggesting that if a person is overloaded with work, it may be because he systematically takes too much time to do a job. This can be applied to all areas of work within general practice. The quality of work is not necessarily related to the time taken to complete a task: one member of staff may achieve the same result in less time than another. However, patient care often involves subjective assessment and is therefore difficult to quantify. The word 'routine' describes an established course or procedure (Adair, 1988b). Routines can become mechanical, inflexible, uninspired and therefore more time consuming. Because they are habitual, they tend to escape close scrutiny.

> **Activity 2.8: Write down instances when you have taken longer to do a task than the time allocated. Make notes on why this might have occurred. Examples may include: (a) insufficient time initially being allocated for the procedure; (b) completing a more thorough assessment of the patient; (c) undertaking other tasks unrelated to the initial consultation, for example hypertension screening or updating immunizations; and (d) chatting to your patient. List ways in which you could have improved your efficiency and effectiveness.**

Good organization involves planning (Box 2.6), delegation and communication. These issues are closely linked and difficult to separate.

Box 2.6: Planning

Good planning will help to:

- reduce time pressure
- allow creative time (thinking how to set up a task)
- allow preparatory time for organizing resources
- permit productive time, when unscheduled jobs are kept to a minimum and deadlines met

---

Planning

Torrington and Weightman (1994) offer a simple method of recording and analysing current workload to identify areas where inefficiencies lie. Daily activities are recorded for a specified period, at the end of which the record is analysed to identify time spent on particular activities and to propose specific actions to improve efficiency. Although this may appear to be a time-wasting exercise, the record may highlight inappropriate workload or poor delegation. Data are then available to support a request for clerical support, more nursing hours or better skill mix.

Having identified current working practice, it is essential to have a daily diary (Figure 2.6) and a weekly or annual programme to reduce time pressures and allow time for planning.

8.30 am	Read mail – bin irrelevant items, put journals to one side to read, save mail to answer at end of shift Prepare for day's planned work
8.40 am	Start appointments/patient care
10.20 am	Tidy treatment area
10.30 am	Break
10.40 am	Continue patient care
12.00 am	Tidy treatment area, check stock/re-order Take/make telephone calls Liaise with other disciplines Reply to mail General administration/audit/write standards/read journal/see representatives
1.00 pm	Lunch

Figure 2.6: Example of planned time management.

Individual health needs are not predictable, and it is therefore difficult to allocate to a task a set time limit. If a daily planner is not working well, you may be trying to accomplish too much in a day. The day should be planned to include time for administrative tasks (Box 2.7). If time is used productively, unscheduled jobs are kept to a minimum and deadlines can be met. The quality of time matters more than the quantity of time.

Deskmanship is a skill to be developed. A desk should be clear of all paper except the specific job in hand (Adair, 1988b). This allows concentration on one task at a time and reduces the frustration and tension that accompany the feeling of being 'snowed under'. A well-organized desk reduces time spent searching for important papers or patient notes, continuation cards or paper clips.

Box 2.7: Examples of administration tasks

- Reading and answering mail
- Writing referral letters
- Liaising with colleagues
- Making telephone calls
- Seeing representatives
- Stocking and ordering
- Computer work
- Writing aims and objectives/standards/audit
- Professional development, e.g. reading journals

For efficiency, paper should be handled only once; read and reply, read and file, or read and dispose. Circulars and important articles can be filed systematically for access by the practice team.

If administrative time is double-booked with general nursing duties, it may be necessary to liaise with the practice manager to remedy the situation. Only 60 per cent of the day should be programmed. This allows time to deal with unexpected situations or emergencies (crises).

Regular morning, lunch and afternoon breaks should be planned into the day to regenerate staff, who will then work better (Godefroy and Clark, 1990).

The development of a proactive approach to health, such as health promotion and research, demands planned time. Martin (1995) recommends five tools to help nurses find time for research: make research a priority, collaborate with others, break projects into manageable parts, structure work so that one outcome is research, and identify resources.

Prioritizing

All tasks should be prioritized (Box 2.8), but it is essential in prioritizing not to procrastinate. Procrastination is described as putting off doing something that should be done – intentionally, habitually and reprehensibly (Adair, 1988b). Resolve not to postpone what is ready to be done today. Deal with mail on a daily basis: reply to letters, read the journals, read and file important circulars, and bin the rubbish. Writing standards may also be a task that is deferred. Unfortunately, these issues will eventually have to be addressed.

Box 2.8: Prioritizing

- Must do (top priority) – tasks that must be completed or programmed during the day, e.g. booked appointments
- Should do (medium priority) – time element not so important, e.g ordering stocks, liaising with other disciplines, writing standards, audit
- Could do today, or defer until tomorrow (low priority) – non-essential activities, e.g. tidying cupboards

---

Activity 2.9: Consider a normal week. Place your regular tasks in one of the three categories of priority. Note any changes you can make to improve your workload.

Crisis intervention

Emergencies (crises) are a common hazard in general practice. Walk-in casualties require priority care. It is essential to take five minutes to regain one's calm, review the list of tasks and re-evaluate the priorities (Godefroy and Clark, 1990). You can learn from a critical experience and prepare for future crises. The daily diary should allow time for crisis intervention.

Work overload

Professionals experience stress because of too much work (work overload), whereas other workers are more likely to suffer from insufficient work (work underload) (Blyton et al., 1989). Work underload is unlikely to apply to any practice staff in the foreseeable future. The worst offenders for time wasting are often those who seem to be working hardest and longest; they do not manage their time well.

Possible causes of work overload for practice nurses include:

- an increase in the practice population – new patient checks;
- health promotion requirements (and paperwork);
- the extended role of the nurse, including family planning, chronic disease management, cervical cytology;
- anything else the general practitioner wishes to delegate;
- covering for colleagues who are sick, on leave or taking study days;
- insufficient nursing hours for the practice population.

Effectiveness at work depends on knowing what not to do (Professional Development, 1994). A nurse who is asked to do more tasks than one can realistically be expected to complete has the right to say 'no'. Learn to decline with tact and firmness. Flexibility is essential: no one should be a slave to a planned daily programme.

Delegation

Work is usually generated by delegation from above and below (Figure 2.7). The most efficient method of time management is through delegation to the person who will be working at his optimum level (Godefroy and Clark, 1990). Delegation saves time and develops subordinates.

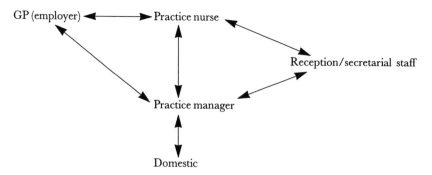

Figure 2.7: Flowchart for delegation.

Delegation implies transferring initiative and authority to another person to perform an agreed task (Adair, 1988b). The subordinate must have the necessary competence for the role, together with a willingness to accept it. Delegation is not the abdication of a role, as some degree of control is still necessary. Delegation is a great motivator. It enriches jobs, improves performance and raises morale.

Time should be spent considering which tasks can be delegated up and down the hierarchy. The ordering of health promotion literature, stock checks and inputting computer data can be delegated to non-nursing staff.

It may not be appropriate for untrained staff to weigh patients and undertake urinalysis; these procedures necessitate an understanding of the results. However, unqualifed staff can be trained to undertake certain tasks that will release time for qualified nurses to utilize their skills (skill mix).

Doctors often delegate down to nurses, who should be appropriately trained to undertake specific tasks in order to ensure personal professional accountability.

It could be argued that it is inappropriate to delegate child immunization sessions to practice nurses who have no experience or training in child abuse or child health. Readers may wish to consider their current position with regard to child immunization, the administration of psychiatric medication and the administration of family planning treatments.

Communication

Good communication allows each team member to know precisely what is required of him or her. Clear instructions for deadlines prevent misunderstandings. Communication may be oral, written or both. Message books are useful but must not be used to the exclusion of face-to-face contacts.

It can be difficult to ask someone to leave after a meeting, whether formal or informal. Meeting in someone else's office allows the visitor to determine when to leave. Talkative people, including pharmaceutical representatives, are best given an appointment just before lunch: this keeps the meeting short. However, lunch meetings with visitors and colleagues may be a productive use of time.

Meetings

It is necessary to spend time to save time. Planning, organizing and evaluating teamwork are essential elements of good practice. Regular efficiently chaired practice meetings allow plans to be formulated and evaluated. However, meetings are potential time-wasters. An agenda should always be circulated prior to the meeting in order to increase efficiency. The length of time for the meeting should be specified and adhered to. Multidisciplinary meetings allow the feedback of information and problems and solutions discussed.

Nurse meetings are essential for sharing knowledge and planning standards. Time should be allocated for this purpose.

Reducing interruptions

Much of a planned day may be interrupted. These interruptions may be classed as 'good' or 'bad', but they often cannot be eliminated. A 'good' interruption may be a request to undertake a task for which the nurse is paid, such as wound care or vaccinations. A 'bad' interruption may be an inappropriate telephone call.

Interruptions can be reduced by having a set time for taking calls and seeing visitors (pharmaceutical representatives or clinical specialists) (Pedler et al., 1986). If a patient or caller has no appointment, it is advisable set a time limit: 'I have five minutes. Will that do, or would you rather fix a time later?'

Incoming telephone calls should be restricted to specified times, such as coffee breaks or the end of surgery, to avoid interrupting a consultation. Emergency calls are an exception, and all staff should be aware of which conditions constitute an urgent call. Details of non-urgent calls could be taken by the reception staff and dealt with at a more appropriate time. Care must be taken by all staff to minimize interruptions.

The worst person for interrupting you is yourself (Adair, 1988b). This includes breaks for making coffee, dropping one project for another or stopping work for a chat. These actions must be balanced between time-wasting and regenerative breaks.

What about the patient's time?

It must not be forgotten that patients also have to manage their time. Their other commitments may include work, other medical appointments and family or social commitments. Although they like to be seen quickly for their appointments, patients like the doctor or nurse to have plenty of time to listen to their problems (Pritchard et al., 1986). If the nurse runs behind with her appointments, people usually respond well to a simple 'I'm sorry to have kept you waiting' and a thorough consultation. The nurse who regularly falls behind with booked appointments may need to reassess her time management.

Time spent in the initial patient consultation may reduce the number of subsequent consultations. However, for those patients who never seem to want to go home, a pre-arranged telephone call from a colleague can hasten the conclusion of an overlong consultation.

Summary

It is important to remember that time is a precious commodity for both patient and nurse. Pritchard et al. (1986) acknowledge the uncertainty and difficulty of planning in general practice, where staff sickness and crisis management are unavoidable. Box 2.9 summarizes effective time management in general practice (Edwards, 1994). Training in time management for all staff is essential to improve communication and the appreciation of each team member's role.

Box 2.9: Methods of achieving effective time management (Edwards, 1994)

- Recognition that patients also have to manage their time
- Planning holidays and study leave in advance to spread the workload as evenly as possible
- A daily diary, with specified appointments and duties
- Programming administration time into the day; to include time for professional development
- Appropriate delegation
- Regular breaks to regenerate staff
- Flexibility to deal with crises

Jones (1996) quotes the scenario of a nurse who gave a rubella vaccine to a pregnant woman. Ultimately, the nurse is professionally accountable for her actions, but improved communication between herself and the reception staff might have prevented the incident.

Improved efficiency through delegation and communication will reduce stress, enhance working conditions and raise morale. Good administrative skills reduce the muddle that makes work and wastes time.

Nurses who are interested in research will plan their time to read, prepare and undertake study within their working day. Over-preoccupation with time is not an attractive quality. Live one day at a time. You cannot change what happened yesterday, but you can make tomorrow better by living well today (Adair, 1988b).

Key points:

1. Time is a precious resource for both staff and patients.
2. Good organization involves planning, delegation and communication.

3. Good time management should provide time for professional development, including research.
4. Don't be a slave to time.

References

Adair J (1988a) Effective Leadership. London: Pan.

Adair J (1988b) Effective Time Management. How To Save Time and Spend it Wisely. London: Pan.

Attree M (1993) An analysis of the concept 'quality' as it relates to contemporary nursing care. International Journal of Nursing Studies 30(4): 355–69.

Berger JT, Rosner F (1996) The ethics of practice guidelines. Archives of Internal Medicine 156: 2051–6.

Blyton P, Hassard J, Hill S, Starkey K (1989) Time, Work and Organisation. London: Routledge.

Buchanan DA, Huczynski AA (1985) Organizational Behaviour: An Introductory Text. Hemel Hempstead: Prentice Hall.

Cohen P (1996) Market logic fragments health visiting service. Health Visitor 69(1): 5.

Department of Health (1987) Promoting Better Health. London: HMSO.

Department of Health (1989) Working for Patients: The Health Service Caring for the 1990s. London: HMSO.

Department of Health (1994) The Challenges for Nursing and Midwifery in the 21st Century: The Heathrow Debate. London: HMSO.

Donabedian A (1988) The quality of care. How can it be assessed? Journal of the American Medical Association 260(12): 1743–8.

Dorrell S (1996) Primary Care: The Future. London: NHSE.

Drucker P (1974) New templates for today's organisations. In Buchanan DA, Huczynski AA (Eds) (1985) Organizational Behaviour: An Introductory Text. Hemel Hempstead: Prentice Hall.

Edwards M (1994) Time to go home. Practice Nursing (22 March – 4 April): 20–2.

Edwards M (1996) Assessing quality of general practice care. Practice Nurse 12(1): 33–5, 37.

Ellis R, Whittington D (1993) Quality Assurance in Health Care. A Handbook. London: Edward Arnold.

Godefroy C, Clark J (1990) The Complete Time Management System. London: Judy Piatkus.

Grol R (1993) Development of guidelines for general practice. British Journal of General Practice 43: 146–51.

Handy C (1991) The Age of Unreason, 2nd Edn. London: Business Ltd.

Handy C (1993) Understanding Organisations, 4th Edn. Harmondsworth: Penguin.

Jones M (1996) Accountability in Practice. A Guide to Professional Responsibility for Nurses in General Practice. Salisbury: Quay Books.

Lawley L (1997) Nurse practitioners, do we need them? West Midlands Journal of Primary Care 1: 40–3.

Luft S (1994) The dynamics of practice nursing. In Luft S, Smith M (Eds) Nursing in General Practice. London: Chapman & Hall.

Macgregor Burns J (1978) Leadership. New York: Harper & Row.

Martin PA (1995) Ask an expert. Finding time for research. Applied Nursing Research 8(3): 151–3.

Maslow AH (1943) A theory of human motivation. In Buchanan DA, Huczynski AA (1985) Organizational Behaviour: An Introductory Text. Hemel Hempstead: Prentice Hall.

National Health Service Executive (1996) Choice and Opportunity. Primary Care: The Future. London: Stationery Office.

National Health Service Management Executive (1993) New World, New Opportunities: Nursing in Primary Health Care. London: NHSME.

Pedler M, Burgoyne J, Baydell T (1986) Manager's Guide to Self-development. Maidenhead: McGraw-Hill.

Perry A, Rowe M (1993) Beating time. Nursing Times 89(13): 32–4.

Peters DA (1995) Outcomes: the mainstay of a framework for quality care. Journal of Nursing Care Quality 10(1): 61–9.

Pritchard P, Low K, Whalen M (1986) Management in General Practice. Oxford: Oxford University Press.

Professional Development (1994) Time management. Revision notes. Nursing Times 90(20): Unit 6, Part3/3, p. 10.

Ranade W (1994) A Future for the NHS? Health Care in the 1990's. London: Longman.

Rix A, Elwyn GJ (1996) Managing health visitors in general practice. Health Visitor 69(1): 15–16.

Sale D (1996) Quality Assurance for Nurses and Other Members of the Health Care Team, 2nd Edn. Basingstoke: Macmillan.

Schein EH (1986) Organisational Culture and Leadership. San Francisco: Jossey Bass.

Strong P, Robinson J (1990) The NHS under New Management. Milton Keynes: Open University Press.

Torrington D, Weightman J (1989) Effective Management: People and Organisations. London: Prentice Hall.

Torrington D, Weightman J (1994) Effective Management 2nd ed. London: Prentice Hall.

Townsend P, Whitehead M, Davidson N (1992) Inequalities of Health. London: Penguin.

United Kingdom Central Council for Nursing, Midwifery and Health Visiting (1996) Guidelines for Professional Practice. London: UKCC.

Further reading

Handy C (1993) Understanding Organisations, 4th Edn. Harmondsworth: Penguin. This book contains an adaptation of a useful self-evaluation question-naire (Harrison's Inventory) to help you to assess the values and styles of your organization and how these equate with your own.

Kemp N, Richardson E (1990) Quality Assurance in Nursing Practice. Oxford: Butterworth-Heinemann.

Miles A, Lugon M (Eds) Effective Clinical Practice. London: Blackwell Science.

Ovretveit J (1992) Health Service Quality, an Introduction to Quality Methods for Health Services. London: Blackwell Scientific.

Royal College of Nursing (1991) Standards of Care in Practice Nursing. London:Scutari Projects.

Scott CD, Jaffe DT (1990) Managing Organisational Change. London: Kogan Page. This book describes the transition grid and the force-field analysis first suggested by Kurt Lewin in 1947. These are simple to apply and provide a practical framework for action.

Chapter 3
Infection control

Mandy Beaumont and Helen Jenkinson

Infection control should be an accepted part of the practice nurse's role. Research quoted in this chapter, however, suggests that nurses' knowledge of infection control is poor. This chapter has been written to help practice nurses to assess their current practice and identify areas in which improvements can be made. Although the specific control of wound infection has not been included in this chapter, many of the recommended guidelines are relevant.

It is accepted that changing a practice routine and obtaining the resources to change policy can be very difficult for some people. Small changes will lead to an overall improvement in infection control; many small changes will make a significant difference. Readers who currently meet all the recommendations are to be commended!

> Does not the popular idea of infection involve that people should take greater care of themselves than of the patient? That for instance it is safer to not to be too much with the patient, not to attend too much to his wants? Perhaps the best illustration of the utter absurdity of this view of duty in attending on infectious diseases is afforded by what was very recently the practice, if it is not so even now, in some of the European Lazarets – in which the plague-patient used to be condemned to the horrors of filth, over-crowding, and want of ventilation, while the medical attendant was ordered to examine the patient's tongue through an opera glass and to toss him a lancet to open his abscesses with, ... True nursing ignores infection except to prevent it ... Wise and humane management of the patient is the best safe guard against infection. (Nightingale, 1859)

Introduction

Communicability is a factor that differentiates infection from non-infectious diseases. The transmission of pathogenic organisms to other people, directly or indirectly, may lead to an epidemic. Many infections are preventable by hygiene measures, by vaccines or by the wise use of drugs (chemoprophylaxis).

Infection control is a system of methods by which patients are protected from infection (Ayliffe et al., 1992) and is fundamental to the provision of a safe environment and quality care for patients. Infection control has been practised in a variety of fragmented forms since 1850 when Semmelweiss noted varying mortality rates from puerperal sepsis in deliveries undertaken by different staff groups.

There is evidence that the standard of infection control knowledge amongst general nurses is poor (Gould, 1995). Studies have shown that provision for good infection control practice within general practice is poor (Hoffman et al., 1988; Foy et al., 1990; Morgan et al., 1990).

With the shift in emphasis from secondary to primary health care provision, and with increasing numbers of minor surgical interventions, it is essential that infection control becomes a priority within the general practice arena.

The reasons for a reduction of disease in the twentieth century

There have been successes in the control of communicable disease in the past century, although credit is due more to improvements in nutrition and living conditions than immunization and antibiotics. Factors that have influenced the patterns of infection developed in countries during the past two decades are summarized in Box 3.1.

Box 3.1: Factors influencing patterns of infection

- Microbial resistance
- Immune suppression
- Foreign travel
- Sexual behaviour
- Drug addiction
- Discovery of new microbes
- Changes in animal husbandry
- Food production
- Availability/uptake of vaccines
- Improved standard of living

Pathology of infection

Disease due to infection is the result of the interaction between micro-organisms and the defence mechanisms of the body.

Source and spread

Infection that may originate from the patient (autogenous) is usually from the skin, nasopharynx or bowel. Outside (exogenous) sources include another person who is suffering from infection or carrying pathogenic micro-organisms. Carriers are usually healthy and may harbour the organism in their throat (e.g. diphtheria), bowel (e.g. salmonella) or blood (e.g. hepatitis B or HIV). Reservoirs of infection other than human ones include:

- water – cholera;
- milk – tuberculosis;
- food – botulism;
- animals – rabies;
- birds – psittacosis;
- soil and water – Legionnaires' disease.

Definitions

The *incubation period* is the time between the invasion of the tissues by pathogens and the appearance of clinical features of acute illness.

The *period of infectivity* is the period of time that the patient is infectious to others.

Bacteraemia is the presence of living micro-organisms in the blood, which can occur in people without causing symptoms.

Septicaemia occurs when organisms enter the bloodstream, actively multiply and produce toxins. Organisms causing septicaemia may originate from one of the areas of the body that are normally colonized by micro-organisms, for example skin, large bowel and genital tract, or originate from organs such as the kidney or liver.

Toxaemia implies a concentration of bacterial toxins in the blood.

Acute illness is the stage at which the disease reaches its full intensity.

Hand-washing

Hand-washing describes a process that removes potentially pathogenic organisms from the hands, the aim of which is to prevent the hands becoming a vehicle for cross-infection.

In order to reduce the transmission of infection, it is vital that the hands of the health care worker are clean and washed regularly, and that the hand-washing technique is of a high standard. In order to prevent the spread of infection, practice nurses need to be prepared to challenge their own hand-washing technique and that of their colleagues. Types of hand-washing are summarized in Table 3.1.

Table 3.1: Types of hand-washing

Type	Materials	When used
Social	Soap and water	After visiting the toilet and before starting work, going home or attending the next patient
Hygienic	Medicated soap, e.g. chlorhexidine	Before aseptic technique and after contact with an infected patient
Surgical	Chlorhexidine, povidone iodine	Prior to surgical intervention to kill transient organisms and a substantial number of resident organisms

The importance of hand-washing as a means of preventing cross-infection should be the first task a student nurse learns. However, despite knowledge, training and continuing education, nurses do not always wash their hands as often, or as well, as they should.

Taylor (1978) found that some nurses thought that there was no risk of cross-infection if they had not touched a soiled object or their hands did not look dirty. It is hoped that, if Taylor's research were conducted today, the results might be a little more favourable and there would have been an improvement in the hand-washing technique of all health care workers.

In the primary health care setting, there are many procedures undertaken in one area. It is very rare for practice premises to allow separate clinical rooms for minor surgery, well-men clinics and wound dressing. It is therefore vital that hand-washing facilities are conveniently located throughout the clinical area.

Resources

The resources used for hand-washing must not create a cross-infection hazard. Bowell (1992) states that poorly cleaned and maintained hand-basins and soap dispensers may create a cross-infection risk. The resources that are available must be well maintained and, if broken, damaged or the practice nurse considers that they are a cross-infection risk, the equipment must be replaced. Advice about replacing equipment can be sought from the community infection control nurse.

Hand-washing technique

The hand-washing technique described in Box 3.2 is based on a procedure described by Ayliffe et al. (1992) and is recommended as the most effective method of decontaminating hands.

Box 3.2: Recommended hand-washing technique (Ayliffe et al., 1992)

1. Sufficient soap (bar or liquid) should be applied to the hands to obtain a good lather. Hand-washing or disinfecting technique, regardless of the product selected, must ensure that no area of skin surface is missed during the procedure.

RUB THE HANDS:
2. palm to palm;
3. right palm over left dorsum, and left palm over right dorsum;
4. palm to palm, fingers interlaced;
5. backs of fingers to opposing palms with fingers interlocked;
6. rotational rubbing of right thumb clasped in left palm and vice versa;
7. rotational rubbing, backwards and forwards with the clasped fingers of right hand in left palm and vice versa.

When to wash the hands

Hand-washing after each patient contact is essential. Effective hand-washing is the single most important infection control measure. Larson and Killien (1982) state that there are five components that together comprise quality hand-washing. These are technique, agent used, appropriateness, duration and frequency.

For hand-washing in minor surgery, see Box 3.3. A separate deep sink is recommended for the washing of instruments.

Drying hands

Following washing, hands should then be thoroughly rinsed under running water for a further 10–15 seconds and dried, preferably with a paper towel. The friction caused by rubbing and rinsing the hands, coupled with the rough action of paper towels, should physically remove micro-organisms (Gould and Ream, 1993).

Box 3.3: Hand-washing for minor surgery

- The hand-washing sink should be fitted with an elbow-operated mixer tap.
- There should be a supply of soap and disposable paper towels next to the sink.
- If nailbrushes are used, they should be single use and sterile; repeated scrubbing with nailbrushes will damage the skin and may be associated with an increase in the number of resident bacteria.
- Before the first surgical case, the hands and forearms should be washed thoroughly with soap and water for 2 minutes.

Note that:
- Antiseptic detergent hand-wash preparations are usually chlorhexidine or iodine based.
- Surgical hand disinfection should be carried out prior to performing any minor surgery.

Wearing gloves

In the past, health care workers have been encouraged to reduce the use of protective clothing, in the belief that it demonstrated a barrier to communication. However, with the advent of Human Immunodeficiency Virus (HIV) in the early 1980s, the use of protective clothing has become common practice for many nurses in the clinical area.

The Department of Health (UK Health Department, 1990) recommended that all health care workers should adopt universal precautions (Box 3.4) when caring for clients.

Box 3.4: Universal precautions

- Apply good basic hygiene practices with regular hand-washing
- Cover existing wounds or skin lesions with waterproof dressings
- Avoid invasive procedures if suffering from chronic skin lesions on the hands
- Avoid contamination of person by appropriate use of protective clothing
- Protect mucous membranes of eyes, mouth and nose from blood splashes
- Prevent puncture wounds, cuts and abrasions in the presence of blood
- Avoid sharps usage wherever possible
- Institute approved procedures for the disinfection and sterilization of instruments and equipment
- Clear up spillages of blood and other body fluids promptly, and disinfect surfaces
- Institute a procedure for the safe disposal of contaminated waste

The interpretation of universal precautions and the use of personal protective equipment (PPE) has meant that gloves tend to be overused. However, the debate of when to wear gloves and when not to wear gloves is coupled with 'which glove to wear' for which procedure. Gloves should be used:

• to prevent hands becoming contaminated;
• to prevent the transfer of organisms already present on the skin and to minimize cross-infection, thereby protecting the nurse and the client.

The decision to wear gloves rests with the practitioner. The practice nurse has to make an informed choice about glove usage, remembering that the protection of both client and health care worker is vital.

Disposable gloves should be worn:

• to protect the user while handling infectious material, i.e. blood, faeces and urine;
• to protect the client from transient micro-organisms.

Plastic aprons and disposable gloves should be worn when the practitioner expects contact with blood or body fluids. PPE is designed to provide a barrier between the patient and the health care worker to protect both from the transmission of infection. It is not intended that wearing gloves should replace hand-washing: they should be employed in addition to thorough hand-washing and drying.

Sharps disposal

Needles should not be resheathed. The syringe and needle should be discarded as one unit into a recommended sharps container, which must comply with BS7320 and UN3291; sharps must never be left to be disposed of by someone else. Sharps containers should be sealed and labelled with the name of the practice and discarded when they are no more than three-quarters full (never being placed in a yellow bag). All sharps must be disposed of by incineration. Sharps boxes in use should be positioned out of reach of patients.

Inoculation injury guidelines are outlined in Box 3.5.

Box 3.5: Inoculation injury guidelines

First aid
- Stop what you are doing and attend the injury
- Bleed the area
- Always wash the injured area with soap and running water
- Cover with a waterproof dressing

Report the incident
- A record of the whole incident must be made and kept. This should include the names of those involved
- Depending on the circumstances of the incident and those involved, it may be necessary to take a blood sample from the individual concerned. Testing of blood is only undertaken following consent and counselling. To obtain further information on what action to take, contact the consultant in public health medicine or the community infection control nurse
- It is advisable that staff contact their general practitioner or the public health department to see whether further action is required even if the staff member has received immunization against hepatitis B

Minor surgery in general practice

Minor surgical operations have been part of general practice for many years. Prior to 1990 and the general practitioner minor surgery scheme, approximately 25 per cent of general practitioners carried out minor surgical procedures in their practices. This number has now increased to approximately 75 per cent. Today, minor surgery is part of everyday life for the practice nurse, and her role in minor surgery is vital. The outcome of the procedure depends upon the skill of the doctor and the nursing support, alongside the implementation of good infection control procedures.

The clinical room

Clean and dirty areas should be clearly defined to reduce the risk of cross-infection (Table 3.2). All surfaces should be impermeable and easy to clean.

Appropriate protective clothing (i.e. a plastic apron and household gloves) should be worn during all cleaning procedures. Cleaning equipment such as mops and cloths should be used only in the clinical area. Colour coding of the equipment may be a useful way of ensuring that clinical cleaning equipment is not used in other areas of the practice.

Table 3.2: Infection control in the clinical room

Fixture	Type	Method of cleaning
Floors	Vinyl with welded seams	Cleaned daily at the end of each day or session using detergent and water
Walls	Painted with oil-based paint	Cleaned on a 6-monthly basis or when visibly soiled
Radiators	Painted with oil-based paint	Cleaned on a 6-monthly basis or when visibly soiled
Examination lights	Easy to clean to prevent build-up of dust	Clean using a damp cloth soaked in water and detergent at the end of each session
Mechanical ventilation, i.e. electric extractor fan	Easy to clean	Inspect on monthly basis and clean on 3-monthly basis to prevent build-up of dust
Suction tubing	Should be disposable	Disposable
Suction jar	Easy to clean	Contents of the jar should be discarded carefully down the sluice or toilet to prevent the production of aerosols. The jar should be washed in hot soapy water and stored dry
Cubicle curtains	Easy to clean	Cleaned every 6 months or when visibly soiled

Equipment

Disposable paper sheeting should be used for examination and operating couches. Blankets, if used, should be washed on a weekly basis
and when visibly soiled. Ideally, all linen should be laundered by an
outside contractor. If it is to be laundered on site, local advice can be
obtained from the infection control nurse.

Hand-washing is described in Box 3.3.

Preparing the patient

The aim of disinfecting skin sites prior to surgery is to remove and
reduce the number of resistant bacteria. The preparation product
used should be fast acting and have a prolonged antibacterial effect,
although skin reactions may occur with some products. The skin

cleansing solution should be applied liberally to the site and surrounding area, and then allowed to dry. Skin disinfection should be carried out immediately prior to surgery.

Personal protective equipment

The practice nurse assisting in minor surgical procedures should wear a disposable plastic apron. Sterile latex gloves should be used for any procedure involving contact with normally sterile areas of the body. Gloves and aprons should be disposed of as clinical waste.

Clinical waste

Clinical waste should always be placed in a foot-operated waste bin. Yellow clinical waste bags should be removed at the end of each session or day and placed in the designated holding area for clinical waste (see below).

Protection of staff and patients

Patient safety must be safeguarded at all times. The immunization of staff against hepatitis B is essential, and the practice nurse must comply with Department of Health guidelines on hepatitis B (DoH, 1996).

Disinfection

The decontamination of equipment between patients, especially where there is a high risk of spread of infection, is the responsibility of the practice nurse. Non-adherence to safe practice will jeopardize the standard of care delivered to the patient and will therefore be a direct violation of the UKCC Code of Conduct for nurses (see Chapter 1).

All disinfectants are potentially hazardous and must be used with caution. For example, hypochlorites corrode metals and bleach fabrics. Hypochlorite concentration is measured in parts per million (ppm) available chlorine. It is recommended that spills of blood be disinfected by cleaning with hypochlorite solution. However, as suggested above, there are many surfaces that will be damaged by the use of hypochlorite. All disinfectants should be assessed for risk under the requirement of the Control of Substances Hazardous to Health (COSHH) regulations 1994 (HSE, 1994) and stored in a locked cupboard in accordance with COSHH regulations. Liquid bleach, which is less safe and less convenient than hypochlorite, should be stored in a cool, dark place and used within six months. Fresh solutions of cleaning agents should be made up daily as required.

Spillages of blood and body fluids should be dealt with as described in Table 3.3.

Table 3.3: Spillage guidelines

Any spillage must be cleaned up as soon as possible. Always wear an apron and disposable gloves before handling any body fluids

Type	Method
Urine	Clean with general purpose detergent and dry area thoroughly
Faeces/vomit	Wipe up spillages with disposable paper towels. Clean the area using soap and water, and dry thoroughly
Blood	Use chlorine granules to soak up the blood and wipe up with a paper towel. Wash the area with hot water and detergent

Where waste is non-infected, it can simply be swept or mopped up, rebagged or sluiced away as appropriate. Care must be taken with glass and other sharps.

Sterilization

General practitioners are responsible for the effective operation and maintenance of sterilizing equipment in their practices. However, it is often the practice nurse who is most familiar with the day-to-day workings of the equipment and daily function tests.

With the increase in minor surgery within general practice, it is becoming even more important to ensure that equipment is disinfected and sterilized where appropriate. There appears to be confusion about what equipment needs to be disinfected and/or sterilized in general practice and the responsibilities involved when sterilizing instruments.

It is important that staff understand what they are trying to achieve through cleaning, disinfection and sterilization (Box 3.6). Table 3.4 may help to identify what equipment does and does not need to be sterile at the point of use, or sterilized after use.

Box 3.6: Cleaning, disinfection and sterilization

Cleaning: The removal of organic matter is an essential process prior to disinfection or sterilization. It can usually be achieved using hot water and washing-up liquid. The use of chlorhexidine-based hand-washes to clean instruments is expensive and unnecessary

Disinfection: Process leading to the reduction in number of viable micro-organisms but which may not inactivate bacterial spores and some viruses

Sterilization: The destruction of all viable micro-organisms including bacterial spores

---

Table 3.4: Recommendations for cleaning/sterilizing equipment

Risk	Application	Recommendation
High	Items in contact with a break in the skin or mucous membrane, or introduced into a sterile part of the body; e.g. surgical instruments	These instruments must be sterile at the point of use
Intermediate	Items in contact with intact skin, mucous membranes or body fluids, particularly after use on infected patients or prior to use on immunocompromised patients; e.g. examination specula	These instruments need not be sterile at the point of use but must be sterilized after use
Low	Items in contact with intact skin or mucous membranes or not in contact with the patient; e.g. thermometer or surfaces	Cleaning with general-purpose detergent, e.g. washing-up liquid, or chemical disinfection may be appropriate

The use of chemical disinfectants is strictly governed by the COSHH regulations (HSE, 1994), which contain strict guidelines on the use of chemicals such as glutaraldehyde (Cidex), which can expose staff to serious health risks. Adequate facilities such as fume cupboards and PPE must be available. Staff using Cidex, even under controlled conditions, should have their health monitored by an occupational health department or equivalent.

Of course, there are alternatives to each practice owning a sterilizer. Some practices may use disposable sterile equipment; others make arrangements to send their instruments for sterilization at the local sterile supplies department.

If a practice decides to purchase a sterilizer, a transportable autoclave that fully complies with BS3970 (Parts 1 and 4) 1990 and the relevant European Standard, as well as safety specifications conforming to EN61010 Part 2-041, is recommended at the time of writing. A temperature recorder should be considered where the traceability of records is required. The printout can then be attached to the patient notes.

The sterilizer

The Health Technical Memorandum 2010 (HTM, 1994) is regarded as the authoritative work on sterilization and applies to all bench-top sterilizers; it aims to ensure their efficiency and safety. Proper procedures and maintenance of the machine help to ensure that instruments are sterilized.

The memorandum outlines the responsibilities of those involved in purchasing, buying and maintaining a sterilizer. The management's main responsibility, apart from being ultimately accountable, is to appoint or designate the following individuals.

The user is responsible for the management of the sterilizer, which includes deciding, once the sterilizer has been commissioned, whether it is fit for use. This decision is based on the tests that should be carried out each day or, if the sterilizer is used infrequently, prior to its use. The recommended daily sterilizer check and user test record can be seen in Box 3.7.

The practice also needs to ensure that more thorough maintenance is carried out in accordance with HTM2010. These tests can be carried out by a company qualified to do such work. There should always be a record of all the tests and maintenance that have been carried out on the machine so that the practice is able to demonstrate that the regulations have been complied with. The

---

Box 3.7: Daily sterilizer check
Adapted from HTM 2010 (1994)

1. Wipe out/clean sterilizer chamber
2. Check/clean door seal, in accordance with local procedures/manufacturer's instructions
3. Check/fill water reservoir
4. Run cycle and note:
   - temperature 134°C minimum when sterilizing;
   - pressure 2.2bar minimum when sterilizing;
   - sterilization hold time 3.0-3.5 minutes;
   - total cycle time 15 minutes
5. Visual check for leaks or anything unusual
6. Record number of cycles where possible
7. Complete and sign the user record sheet

In the event of a breakdown, inform the maintenance engineer

Sterilizer user test record

Test	1	2	3	4a	4b	4c	4d	5	6	7
Date	Clean chamber	Check door	Check water	Check 134°C	Check 2.2 bar	Check 3.0–3.5 min hold	Check & time 15 min	Check leaks	Record cycles	Print name
1.1.98	✓	✓	✓	✓	✓	✓	✓	✓	2	A.Non
2.1.98	✓	✓	✓	✓	✓	✓	✓	✓	1	A.Non

above recommendations and published guidance, if followed, will reduce the risk of inadequately sterilized instruments being used. The surgery that follows HTM 2010 will be able to demonstrate that it has done everything that is practicably possible to ensure that the sterilizer is working effectively.

Control of Substances Hazardous to Health regulations

The 1988 COSHH regulations, updated in 1994, cover substances that can cause ill-health to either workers or others exposed to those substances. These include those substances that:

- are used at work: chemicals such as cleaning materials;
- arise from work: fumes and waste products;
- occur naturally: micro-organisms.

COSHH regulations require that hazardous substances are identified in the workplace and procedures implemented to protect staff and visitors to the workplace.

Identification

It is important to identify all materials within the workplace that must comply with the COSHH regulations. These can be identified by their warning label.

Assessment

It is important that the hazard and the risk are assessed. Chemicals, for example, may be flammable or harmful if swallowed, and a risk assessment needs to be completed and recorded which identifies the hazard of each chemical used in the practice.

The hazard is the potential of the substance to cause harm, and the risk is the likelihood that it will cause harm in the actual circumstances of use. For example, there can be a risk from a material that is not particularly hazardous if it is used inappropriately and carelessly, whereas the risk of being harmed by a hazardous substance can be very slight if proper precautions are taken.

Control measures

To prevent exposure, the harmful substance should be substituted, where possible, by a non-harmful substance. The process should be enclosed (controlled) by identifying systems of safe working and the use of PPE.

Monitor

Staff working with chemicals that have been identified as hazardous to health may need occupational health checks and follow-up. Within general practice, it is unlikely that there will be any chemicals that fall into this category unless staff are dealing with glutaraldehyde which is not recommended for use in general practice.

Maintain

A programme of continuing training and education should be available for all staff within general practice. This should include information for non-clinical staff in the handling of specimens of blood or body fluid.

Inform

Staff are encouraged to report any problems that they encounter.

Clinical waste

The five categories of clinical waste are listed in Table 3.5.

The guidelines state that the preferred disposal route for all clinical waste is incineration. Group A and B wastes must be incinerated, but group E waste may be landfilled in sites that have a special clinical waste landfill licence.

Table 3.5: Categories of clinical waste

Group A	All human tissue, including blood, soiled surgical dressings, swabs and other soiled waste from treatment areas
Group B	Discarded syringe needles, cartridges, broken glass and any other contaminated disposable sharp instruments or items
Group C	Microbiological cultures and potentially infectious waste from pathology departments
Group D	Certain pharmaceutical products and chemical wastes
Group E	Items used to dispose of urine, faeces and other bodily excretions or secretions not falling within Group A wastes

Segregation

Group A waste must be disposed of in a yellow bag marked 'Clinical waste for incineration only' or with equivalent wording. Group E waste may also be disposed of in these bags. Group B waste (sharps) must be discarded safely into sharps bins that conform to the British Standard 7320 and the UN3291, which will be clearly marked on the box. The BS7320 and UN3291 set standards regarding the design of the box to ensure that sharps placed into the box are rendered safe and that the box will not split or allow the needle to penetrate the side, as well as to prevent needles being taken out of the box. Group E waste that can be landfilled is discarded in yellow bags that have a black stripe on them ('tiger bags'). Group A waste must not be placed into these bags.

Disposal

Clinical waste bags should be placed into foot-operated pedal bins in clinical areas so that staff hands are not contaminated when discarding waste. Sharps boxes must be assembled correctly before use; this can be checked by ensuring that all the edges have clicked down. Sharps boxes should be closed and replaced when they are two-thirds full. Clinical waste bags should be sealed when two-thirds full or at the end of the day. If the bag is twisted and the neck taped back on itself, the leakage of contents is prevented. Bags and boxes must be labelled with the name of the general practitioner practice in accordance with the Duty of Care.

Storage

There are strict guidelines surrounding the storage of clinical waste:

• Clinical waste should not be stored for more than one week before collection by a registered company. If the collection day falls on a holiday, the waste should be collected as soon after that date as possible.
• The storage area should be easy to clean and should be cleaned regularly.
• Spillages should be cleaned up immediately.
• The clinical waste bags must be stored away from the public and must be locked and inaccessible to unauthorized persons and vermin. 'Clinibins' are now available for the storage of full clinical waste bags. They are made of plastic and can be padlocked to a wall, with the lid padlocked shut to protect the contents.

Safe handling

Staff who deal with clinical waste bags should be taught how to handle them safely. Clinical waste bags should be carried by the neck of the bag away from the body and should not be thrown around. Staff should be provided with suitable protective clothing, i.e. plastic apron and household gloves, when handling clinical waste.

Spillage

The guidelines for dealing with spillage are outlined in Table 3.3 (p. 73).

Sharps injury

The Health Service Advisory Committee recommends that staff know how to deal with a sharps injury to either themselves or colleagues. It is important that each practice is aware of the local sharps injury policy. Box 3.5 above contains inoculation injury guidelines.

A checklist (Box 3.8) may help practices to identify whether they comply with the regulations.

Vaccine storage

The cold chain and its maintenance is an important component of any immunization programme. In studies conducted by the World Health Organization, a low potency of vaccines was identified, among other factors, as one of the major factors affecting seroconversion. Immunization gives rise to immunity, and immunity of population leads to disease reduction. However, immunity can result only from the use of active and effective vaccines.

Adu et al. (1996) describe active and effective vaccines as needing four essential elements within the cold chain in order to sustain potency:

- equipment – well-insulated cool boxes, designated well-maintained fridges and a maximum/minimum thermometer;
- manpower – trained staff;
- transportation – appropriate vehicles and speed;
- vaccines – quality of the vaccine at the time of administration.

A break in the cold chain at any of these points has long been associated with a low seroconversion rate in vaccine programmes.

Box 3.8: The following checklist may help practices to identify whether they comply with the regulations (adapted from the audit tool created by the West Midlands Infection Control Nurses Association, with permission).

	YES	NO
1. Waste is segregated correctly		
Household waste is disposed of in black bags	⬭	⬭
Clinical waste is disposed of in yellow bags marked for incineration only	⬭	⬭
Sharps are disposed of in sharps boxes that conform to BS7320 and UN3291	⬭	⬭
2. Disposal		
Pedal bins are available and are in working order	⬭	⬭
Sharps boxes have been assembled correctly	⬭	⬭
Bags have been sealed when two-thirds full	⬭	⬭
Sharps boxes have been closed when two-thirds full	⬭	⬭
Bags and boxes have been labelled with the name of the GP practice	⬭	⬭
3. Storage		
Clinical waste is collected on a weekly basis by a registered company	⬭	⬭
Clinical waste is stored in a locked area, safely away from unauthorized people and pests	⬭	⬭
The storage area is easy to clean and is cleaned regularly	⬭	⬭
4. Handling		
Staff hold the bags by the neck	⬭	⬭
Staff hold the bags away from their bodies	⬭	⬭
Staff do not throw the clinical waste bags into the storage area but always place them carefully on the ground	⬭	⬭
5. Spillage		
Staff can state how to clean up a spillage	⬭	⬭
6. Sharps injury		
Staff know what to do if they or a colleague has a sharps injury	⬭	⬭

If there are any no's, the practice policy needs reviewing.

Guidelines to ensure the correct storage of vaccines are given in Box 3.9.

Box 3.9: Guidelines for storage of vaccines (Department of Health, 1996)

- All vaccines should be stored as recommended by the manufacturer of the vaccine, in order to maintain their potency
- All vaccines should be stored between 2 and 8°C, protected from light and not allowed to freeze
- All vaccine fridges should have a digital minimum/maximum thermometer. A daily record should be kept of the temperature of the fridge. It is recommended that the practice nurse be responsible for the recording of fridge temperatures within the practice
- The fridge should be used only for the storage of vaccines and not for food, drink or specimens
- The vaccine fridge should be defrosted regularly, ensuring that vaccines are stored either in another fridge or in a cool box with cold packs while the fridge is defrosting
- The plug to the fridge should be covered, and a notice should be placed on either the plug or the fridge stating that the fridge should not be turned off at any time
- If the fridge is turned off at any time, the practice nurse should have a list available of all the vaccines stored and their expiry date and date of manufacture
- The frequent opening of the fridge door should be avoided, and recording the temperature of the fridge should be done before the fridge door is opened to remove vaccines
- Ensure a good stock rotation of the vaccines. Shorter-dated vaccines should be put at the front of the fridge to ensure that they are used first
- When transporting vaccines, the temperature should be maintained. Vaccines should always be carried in a cool box, ensuring that the cool pack does not allow the vaccine to freeze
- Vaccines should not touch the side of the fridge or be stored in the door of the fridge
- Do not pack the vaccines too tightly together. The air must circulate around the fridge for the fridge to operate correctly
- Always read the manufacturers' leaflets about the reconstitution and stability of reconstituted vaccines. All unused reconstituted vaccine should be discarded at the end of an immunization session

---

Checklist for the practice nurse

This checklist should be used daily by the appointed responsible person or under his or her direct supervision:

- Maximum/minimum thermometer read, and record temperatures.

- Does the refrigerator need defrosting?
- Warning message is visible: 'This refrigerator contains vaccines and should not be switched off'.
- Refrigerator is packed safely and not overcrowded. Vaccine packs are not touching the sides of the refrigerator or coming into contact with ice.
- Door of refrigerator closes properly.
- Vaccine receipts book is up to date. Vaccine type, date and quantity received, batch number, expiry date, number of doses used, number returned to pharmacy, current stock as number of doses.

Methicillin-resistant *Staphylococcus aureus* MRSA

Staphylococcus aureus is a Gram-positive coccus and is present in the normal nasal flora of 30 per cent of individuals and on the perineum in 15 per cent of people. It can be transiently carried on the hands of health care staff and can survive well in the environment on skin scales and in dust.

Methicillin-resistant *Staph. aureus* (MRSA) strains were first reported in the UK in 1961 and have since been responsible for outbreaks of infection in many parts of the world. There is an epidemic strain that is resistant to the antibiotics that are normally used to treat Staphylococcal infections.

As more and more patients are discharged earlier into the community from hospital, it is vital that practice nurses are aware of changes in the field of infection control and remain up to date with new infections and treatments. Practice nurses need to be able to adapt the knowledge that they have into terminology that the patient will understand.

Some of the questions that the practice nurse is likely to be asked are listed in Box 3.10, with appropriate responses.

Head lice

In recent years, the number of head lice infections appears to have increased. Whether it is increased awareness and revulsion against lice or a genuine increase is uncertain. Parents who find that they or their children have a head lice infection certainly need reassurance. With correct treatment and aftercare, lice can be kept at bay.

It may sometimes be important to put head lice infection into perspective – head lice do not kill; they are a nuisance and no more.

The amount of confusion amongst the population at large and health care professionals may also add to the panic about head lice. Practice nurses need to be aware of the facts about lice to enable them to explain them clearly to their patients and dispel myths and fears. Readers should familiarize themselves with the local policy with regard to head lice, which can be obtained from local public health departments.

Box 3.10: Questions and answers about MRSA (French et al., 1990; Duckworth and Heathcock, 1995; Lambert, 1996)

What is MRSA and what can it do?
MRSA (methicillin-resistant *Staphylococcus aureus*) is a germ that is harmlessly carried by many people on their skin or up their noses without causing an infection. It is carried more easily on skin if that skin is broken or there is a rash, cut or a sore. MRSA may cause wound infections, abscesses or boils

Do I need to stay away from other people?
The patient may have had a recent episode in hospital or have a relative in hospital who has had MRSA and has been isolated. As a rule, patients in hospital are more vulnerable to infection than are the general public. The practice nurse needs to explain that, although MRSA does not cause many problems in the community, patients in hospital with MRSA are isolated to prevent spread of the infection to other hospital patients

Can it be treated?
MRSA can usually be treated successfully using antibiotics different from the ones normally used to treat Staphylococcal infections

Can I still see my family?
People with MRSA in the community should be encouraged to lead a normal life. There is no reason why relatives and friends who are fit and healthy should stay away from patients with MRSA. If relatives are concerned about their own health, they should be advised to speak to their general practitioner or the local infection control nurse. All relatives should be reminded about basic hygiene precautions such as covering cuts and grazes, and attention to hand-washing

How can I stop MRSA spreading?
The main route of transmission is on people's hands so patients should be reminded about the importance of hand-washing and should, if necessary, be taught a good technique

Do I need to take special precautions with my laundry?
No. Laundry that has been in contact with an infected patient should be washed as normal in the hottest wash that the material can tolerate

Facts about lice

Head lice are greyish-brown wingless insects, approximately 2–3 mm long, which live, breed and die on human scalps. They like to stay close to the scalp for warmth, and feed by biting the scalp and sucking blood.

The eggs are grey, the size of a pin head and enclosed in a sac that is 'glued' to the base of the hair near the scalp. After seven days, a young louse (nymph) will hatch and leave the egg shell (nit), which turns white and will grow out with the hair unless physically removed. Head lice are fully mature after 10 days and can live for up to four weeks. The female head louse can lay as many as 10 eggs a day.

Head lice are wingless, cannot fly and do not jump. They need warmth and do not survive away from the scalp. Transmission occurs through close head-to-head contact where the louse walks from one head to another using its claws to hang on to the strands of hair.

Detection of head lice

Parents of school-age children must be advised to check their childrens' hair on a regular basis (preferably weekly) during holidays as well as term time. Apart from what is seen on regular hair checks, other signs that indicate there is an infection are:

- eggs stuck to the hair shaft (which may look like dandruff but cannot be combed out);
- dark, dry powder on the pillows;
- unusually dirty collars;
- undue redness, soreness or itching of the scalp.

Itching may be a sign of infection, but it may take up to three months for the bites to irritate; therefore parents should be encouraged to look for the above signs and not to wait for itching to start. It is far easier, and less painful, to inspect hair that is wet and has conditioner applied. Lice are unable to move quickly in wet hair and are therefore easier to find. The procedure for checking hair is summarized in Box 3.11.

The control of head lice is achieved through a multidisciplinary approach. School nurses provide education in schools through clinics, leaflets and pre-school meetings with parents, at which relevant advice and information is given. Parents may also approach their health visitor, practice nurse, community pharmacist, general practitioner or public health department for further advice.

Box 3.11 Procedure for checking hair for head lice/nits

- Hair should be parted into sections, and each section should be inspected thoroughly before moving on to the next to ensure that the whole head of hair is inspected thoroughly
- Hair should be combed using a plastic detection comb, starting at the root of the hair and combing right to the end
- Hair should be combed over a white surface such as a white sink or a piece of white paper
- Eggs and nits can be observed during combing; they resemble dandruff but cannot be combed out
- Eggs and nits should be removed by hand by squeezing the egg shell between the finger and thumb and drawing it along the hair shaft
- When all the hair has been combed, the detection comb and the white surface should be inspected for lice
- Treatment should be commenced as soon as possible only if live head lice are observed
- The index case must be encouraged to inform close contacts to look for signs of head lice too, and, if these are found, they also need to be treated

---

Treatment

The two forms of treatment currently in use in 1999 are insecticides and the wet combing method. Practice nurses should be aware of the local treatment policy and advise their patients in line with the local public health department guidelines.

Insecticides should be commenced only when live eggs or live head lice are observed as the indiscriminate use of insecticides will lead to resistance.

For further information on head lice, see Maunder (1993) and Burgess (1995, 1996).

Scabies

Scabies has been a common disease for at least 3000 years. It has been associated with being 'dirty' and perhaps promiscuous. The truth, however, is that scabies is caught by prolonged skin-to-skin contact and can affect anyone in the population. Outbreaks of the infection may occur in residential homes and special schools where residents are at particular risk because of the closeness in which staff and residents live.

Facts about scabies

Scabies is an allergic reaction to the presence of *Sarcoptes scabiei*, which is a mite that burrows into the skin in humans. Scabies infection also occurs in other animals, but the scabies mite is specific to each animal.

The egg is laid in the burrow and hatches within 3–5 days. The mature mite lays two or three eggs each day; this can go on for nearly two months. Larvae and nymphs leave the burrow and find protection in hair follicles. The mite burrows into the skin using its legs and mouth parts. The female mite usually spends the rest of her life in the burrow, whereas the immature forms and young adults spend time in the burrows and on the skin surface, from where they can pass to a new host. It is probable that the successful infection of a new host is made possible by the transference of a fertilized female.

The mites can be scratched out by the finger nails during an intensive scratch and can be killed, although sometimes the top of the burrow is scraped away without damage to the mite, which moves out of this position and burrows again.

Transmission

The mite is transferred from one person to another through prolonged skin-to-skin contact. This is most common in families, between health care staff and patients, while holding hands and during intimate contact. The two types of scabies infection, caused by the same mite, are classical scabies and crusted Norwegian or hyperkerotic scabies.

Classical infection

Classical scabies infection is found in healthy people with normal immune systems; the mites are few in number.

A primary infection will normally have no symptoms for up to six weeks following infection. When the patient becomes sensitized to the mite, the symptoms appear, and an inconspicuous, extremely itchy rash will develop. It is not uncommon for patients to scratch themselves until they bleed.

The rash is characteristically found in the webs of the fingers, on the wrists and forearms, in the axillary folds, on the sides of the thorax, around the waist and on the lower quadrants of the buttocks, the insides of the legs and the ankles. The rash is bilaterally symmetrical and may not occur in all these places at once.

Following the primary rash and intense scratching, secondary bacterial infection may occur in the breaks in the skin.

Crusted Norwegian or hyperkerotic scabies

This form of scabies occurs in people whose immune systems can mount no or little defence against the mite. There are an enormous number of mites present on the host, numbering from thousands to hundreds of thousands.

The skin becomes crusty and is often unsightly, but although the patient may feel some discomfort, the rash is not itchy or bilaterally symmetrical and may appear anywhere on the body. Patients with Norwegian scabies are extremely infectious and can often be the cause of outbreaks of classical scabies amongst close contacts.

Treatment of scabies

Usually, an aqueous-based insecticidal lotion is applied to the whole body and left in place for at least 24 hours. A patient who requires treatment should be advised to get someone to help them in order to ensure that the body is thoroughly covered. Attention should be paid to the hands. Nails should be cut short and treatment applied under them using cotton buds. Care should be taken that the lotion does not get into the eyes or on the face.

Oral therapy is available only on a named patient basis and can be used in cases where lotions have proved ineffective.

The close contacts of those who are infected also require treatment, even if they are not displaying symptoms, because of the long incubation period. All close contacts should be identified and everyone should be treated on the same day. Close contacts are:

- those living under the same roof;
- the patient's partner;
- in institutions, clients and care staff who have been in contact with the infected person; in some instances, this will include all staff in the home.

Reasons for prolonged infection

Treatment failure may occur if the lotion has not been applied thoroughly to all parts of the body. The skin should not be washed during the time of treatment. If skin, such as on the hands, needs to be washed, the lotion should be reapplied.

Incomplete contact tracing

It is important that all close contacts are identified and treated at the same time as the infected person, whether or not they are displaying symptoms. This is necessary because of the length of the incubation period.

The role of the practice nurse in the treatment of head lice and scabies

The practice nurse is in an ideal situation to advise patients on contact tracing and how to use the treatments effectively. Equally importantly, she can reassure, educate and dispel myths. Literature should be available, and informative posters displayed at peak times might also be helpful. These can be obtained through the health promotion department or from pharmaceutical companies. (For more information on head lice and scabies, see also Burgess 1995.)

Blood-borne viruses

For the management of patients with blood-borne viruses, the reader is referred to Box 3.4, (page 68), on universal precautions.

Hepatitis B

Hepatitis B virus is present in virtually all body fluids, although only blood, saliva, vaginal fluid and semen have been found to be infectious. The disease is transmitted via permucosal and percutaneous inoculation, perinatally and during sexual intercourse. The average incubation period is 90 days. Hepatitis B occurs globally and in developing countries is more commonly found in intravenous drug users, men who have sex with men, heterosexuals who have multiple partners, and also health care workers. The number of people affected is increasing, and about 600 cases are reported in the UK each year.

The symptoms of the disease (Box 3.12) vary from person to person, ranging from subclinical illness to a fulminating illness that can be fatal. Infants tend to have asymptomatic infections.

Box 3.12: Symptoms of hepatitis

Hepatitis B	*Hepatitis C*
Insidious onset	Subclinical
Anorexia	Mild or severe nausea
Joint pains	Vomiting
Nausea and vomiting	Abdominal discomfort
Abdominal discomfort	Jaundice
Dark urine	Liver failure
Jaundice	Cancer of the liver

The good news is that 90–95 per cent of adults will recover, although 5–10 per cent of adults and 95 per cent of infants with acute infection become long-term carriers. A small number of chronic carriers who are infectious may develop chronic active hepatitis, cirrhosis or liver cancer. Serum blood tests are used to determine the hepatitis B status of an individual. How the test results are interpreted is summarized in Box 3.13.

Box 3.13: Interpreting hepatitis B blood results

HBsAG: Detected in serum, indicating infection, several weeks before and days, weeks or months after the onset of symptoms. The presence of this indicates potential infectivity

HBeAG: The presence of this indicates relatively high infectivity

Anti-HBc: Appears at the onset of the illness and persists indefinitely

Anti-HBc: IgM antibody. Present in high titre during acute infection and then disappears within 6 months (although it can persist in chronic cases). This is a reliable indicator of hepatitis B infection

Anti-HBsAg: The presence of this indicates immunity if it is over 100 i.u.

Carriers are defined as having HBsAg present in their serum for longer than six months

---

Specific immunoglobulin (HBIG) provides passive immunity and can be given to a non-immune person following known exposure to the virus. Hepatitis B is a major concern for health care staff who are exposed to blood and body fluids. The Department of Health recommends that all staff who perform 'exposure-prone procedures' should have their hepatitis B status checked. Staff who do not have immunity can be protected through vaccination, although they must be encouraged to maintain safe working practices.

Health care staff need to be aware of the risks of hepatitis B and know how to protect themselves and their patients (see the universal precautions outlined in Box 3.4, page 68). The reader is referred to Immunisation against Infectious Diseases (Department of Health, 1996) for recommendations and the immunization regime.

Hepatitis D

The signs and symptoms of hepatitis D are similar to those of hepatitis B. Hepatitis D infection is only found where there is an existing hepatitis B infection because the virus-like particle needs the hepatitis B virus in order to infect the cell. Hepatitis B vaccination will therefore help to control the spread of hepatitis D.

The infection may be self-limiting or may develop into a chronic infection. Hepatitis D occurs world wide wherever hepatitis B is found and is transmitted in a similar way to hepatitis B, i.e. via infected blood and some body fluids. The incubation period is about 2–8 weeks, and a person is probably at his peak of infectivity just prior to the onset of the acute illness.

Hepatitis C

Hepatitis C was first identified in 1991 in semen. Prior to 1991, it was grouped amongst the non-A/non-B hepatitis infections. Hepatitis C is found world wide, with humans as the reservoir of infection. The disease is transmitted by the same routes as hepatitis B, although it is probably less infectious. It is thought to be transferred via infected blood, although sexual transmission, sharing contaminated needles and perinatal transmission may account for a small number of cases. The incubation period is approximately 6–9 weeks, although it can range from two weeks to six months.

The symptoms of hepatitis C infection are listed in Box 3.12 above. The virus is also thought to cause other problems, including thyroid abnormalities, polyarthritis and chronic fatigue syndrome.

A national 'look back' exercise in 1995 involved those people who may have contracted hepatitis C via blood transfusion prior to 1991. The Blood Transfusion Centres checked their records to see whether blood donors who had been identified as positive for hepatitis C had given blood prior to 1991. Since September 1991, all blood for transfusion has been screened for hepatitis C; previously there had not been a test available in the UK.

The prevalence of hepatitis C is unknown at the time of writing, and there is no vaccine against it. Newly diagnosed patients require counselling. A cure is not available, although treatment can prove successful and, if taken for 6–12 months, will induce complete (25%) or temporary (50%) remission, at least during treatment.

Human immunodeficiency virus (HIV)

Infection control plays a minor (albeit important) part of caring for patients with HIV and AIDS. The advent of universal precautions ensures that all blood and body fluids are handled safely to protect both staff and patients. The practice nurse must be aware of psychological issues as well as the physical needs that will concern the patient. Information, support and advice can be obtained from local clinical nurse specialists in HIV, and also genito-urinary clinics.

The human immunodeficiency virus was first discovered in 1983, although the acquired immune deficiency syndrome was recognized in 1981 in the USA when there was an increasing number of young men requiring treatment for the previously rare infection *Pneumocystis carinii* pneumonia.

Once the virus enters the body, there is a period of viraemia with or without symptoms, during which the individual is highly infectious. The infection can then remain dormant for many years following the body's production of antibodies, but the infected individual remains potentially infectious to others. There is no vaccine available at present, but new treatments for infected people that inhibit the proliferation of HIV and prevent opportunistic infections are having some success.

Since the discovery of HIV, surveillance has played an important part in discovering more about the disease and about susceptible groups. Monthly summaries of all new cases have been made since 1983. All reporting is voluntary and confidential from clinicians and microbiologists.

In 1996, 2896 new diagnoses of HIV infection in the UK were reported (Hughes, 1997). This is the highest total since 1983, and over half of these patients were less than 35 years old.

The major route of infection in the UK is still through sexual intercourse between men, accounting for over 70 per cent of AIDS cases and over 60 per cent of HIV infection in homosexual or bisexual men. Fifteen per cent of AIDS cases and 19 per cent of HIV infections now lie in the heterosexual group (Hughes, 1997).

Intravenous drug use has made a small but significant contribution to the number of new cases of HIV and AIDS. In Scotland in the late 1980s, there was a real problem amongst intravenous drug users, but, with health promotion and good information, the numbers have reduced from 63 per cent of all HIV infections in Scotland in 1986 to 17 per cent in 1996 (Hughes, 1997). (For more information on blood-borne diseases, see Seymour, 1994; Edwards, 1995; Strassburg and Manns, 1995; Dolan and Hughes, 1997.)

Notifiable diseases

The diagnosing doctor should notify the proper officer, usually based in the public health department, of certain diseases (Table 3.6). It is a legal requirement for which the doctor receives a fee. Notification of disease is an important part of the surveillance and monitoring of different diseases, although it is recognized that there is underreporting.

Table 3.6: Statutorily notifiable diseases

Under the Public Health (Control of Disease) Act 1984

Cholera	Plague
Relapsing fever	Smallpox
Typhus	

Under the Public Health (Infectious Diseases) Regulation 1988

Acute encephalitis	Acute poliomyelitis
Anthrax	Diphtheria
Dysentery (amoebic or bacillary)	Food poisoning
Leprosy	Leptospirosis
Malaria	Measles
Meningitis	Meningococcal septicaemia (without meningitis)
Mumps	Ophthalmia neonatorum
Paratyphoid fever	Rabies
Rubella	Scarlet fever
Tetanus	Tuberculosis
Typhoid fever	Viral hepatitis
Whooping cough	Yellow fever

Local consultants in communicable disease control have the right to add other diseases to the list within their area, but this has to be done through the local law courts. Details of infectivity and the exclusion needs of communicable diseases can be found in the Appendix to this chapter.

Summary

This chapter has briefly summarized areas within general practice where infection control can be influenced by the practice nurse. The infection control guidelines, if followed, will ensure the safety of both patients and staff.

It would be unrealistic to expect immediate major changes in practice policy, but nurses must exercise their accountability to themselves, patients, employers and colleagues by identifying areas in which infection control could be improved. No matter how efficient a general practice considers itself, a closer scrutiny may elicit some unwelcome home truths.

All staff must be aware of infection control policies; this requires a good communication channel to ensure that ancillary staff follow the recommended guidelines (see Chapter 2).

The local public health department and clinical nurse specialists are the main resources for support, literature and data on local infectious diseases (see Chapter 4) and should be approached for further information.

Key points:

1. Infection control is an integral part of cost-effective quality care.
2. All members of the primary health care team, from domestic staff to doctors, must be aware of safe practice.
3. Refer to the infection control nurses for advice and support on any aspects of public health and infection control.

References

Adu FD, Adedeji AA, Essanjs, Odusanya OG (1996) Live viral vaccine potency: an index for assessing the cold chain system. Public Health 110: 325–30.

Ayliffe GAJ, Lowbury EJL, Geddes AM, Williams JD (Eds) (1992) Control of Hospital Infection: A Practical Handbook. London: Chapman & Hall.

Bowell B (1992) A risk to others. Nursing Times 88(4): 38–40.

Burgess IF (1995) Human Lice and their Management. Advances in Parasitology, Vol. 36: Academic Press.

Burgess IF (1996) Management guidelines for lice and scabies. Prescriber 7(9): 87–99.

Department of Health (1996) Immunisation against Infectious Diseases. London: HMSO.

Dolan M, Hughes N (1997) Hepatitis C: a bloody business. Nursing Times 93(45): 71–2.

Duckworth G, Heathcock R (1995) Guidelines on the control of methicillin-resistant *Staphylococcus aureus* in the community. Report of a combined working party of the British Society for Antimicrobial Chemotherapy and the Hospital Infection Society. Journal of Hospital Infection 31: 1–12.

Edwards M (1995) Hepatitis B: the nurse's role. Practice Nursing 6(6): 18–20.

Foy C, Gallagher M, Rhodes T et al. (1990) HIV and measures to control infection in general practice. British Medical Journal of Hospital Infection 3: 29–37.

French GL, Cheng AFB, Ling JML, Mo P, Donnan S (1990) Hong Kong strains of methicillin-resistant and methicillin-sensitive *Staphylococcus aureus* have similar virulence. Journal of Hospital Infection 15(2): 117–25.

Gould D (1995) Infection control: survey to determine nurses' knowledge in a clinical setting. Nursing Standard 9(36): 35–8.

Gould D, Ream M (1993) Assessing nurses' 'hand decontamination performance'. Nursing Times 89(25): 47–9.

Health and Safety Executive (1994) Control of Substances Hazardous to Health Regulations (revised). London: HMSO.

Health Technical Memorandum (1994) The Health Technical Memorandum 2010. Transportable Sterilizers. NHS Estates. Leeds: Agency of the Department of Health.

Hoffman PN, Cooke EM, Larkin DP et al. (1988) Control of infection in general practice: a survey and recommendations. British Medical Journal 297: 34–6.

Hughes G (1997) An overview of the HIV and AIDS epidemic in the United Kingdom. Communicable Disease Report Vol. 7, Review No. 9: 121–2.

Lambert S (1996) Do staff follow guidelines for dealing with MRSA? Nursing Times 92(19): 25–9.

Larson E, Killien M (1982) Factors influencing hand washing behaviour of patient care personnel. American Journal of Infection Control 10(3): 93–9.

Maunder J (1993) How should GPs diagnose and treat headlice? MIMS 16 November: 21–8.

Morgan DR, Lamont TJ, Dawson JD, Booth C (1990) Decontamination of instruments and control of cross infection in general practice. British Medical Journal 300: 1379–80.

Nightingale F (1859) Notes on Nursing: What it is and what it is not. London: Harrison.

Seymour C (1994) Asymptomatic infection with hepatitis C. British Medical Journal 308: 670–1.

Strassburg CP, Manns MP (1995) Autoimmune hepatitis versus viral hepatitis C. Liver 15(5): 225–32.

Taylor LJ (1978) An evaluation of handwashing techniques, Part 2. Nursing Times 74(1): 108–10.

UK Health Departments (1990) Guidance for Clinical Health Care Workers: Protection against Infection with HIV and Hepatitis Viruses. Recommendations of the Expert Advisory group on AIDS. London: HMSO.

Further reading

Allen KW, Humphreys H, Sims-Williams RF (1997) Sterilisation of instruments in general practice: what does it entail? Public Health 111: 115–17.

Atkin K, Hirst M, Lunt N, Parker G (1994) Role and self perceived training needs of nurses employed in general practice: observations from a national census of practice nurses in England and Wales. Journal of Advanced Nursing 20: 46–52.

Benenson A (1995) Control of Communicable Diseases in Man. Washington, DC: American Public Health Association.

British Medical Association (1989) A Code of Practice for Sterilisation of Instruments and Control of Cross Infection. London: BMA.

British Medical Association (1990) A Code of Practice for the Safe Use and Disposal of Sharps. London: BMA.

British Medical Association (1996) Minor Surgery in General Practice. Guidance from the Medical Services Committee and the Royal College of General Practitioners. London: RCGP.

Department of Health (1997) Committee Inquiry into the Future Development of the Public Health Function (Acheson Report). London: HMSO.

Department of Health (1993) Sterilisation, Disinfection and Cleaning of Medical Equipment: Guidance on Decontamination from the Microbiology Advisory Committee to the Department of Health Medical Devices Directorate, Part 1. London: HMSO.

Environmental Protection Act (1990) Waste Management: The Duty of Care: Code of Practice. London: HMSO.

Health and Safety Executive (1992) Personal Protective Equipment at Work. Guidance on Regulations. London: HMSO.

Health Services Advisory Committee (1992) Safe Disposal of Clinical Waste. London: HMSO.

HIV Nursing Society (1994) AIDS/HIV Infection Nursing Guidelines. London: RCN.

Mortimer JY, Evans BG, Goldberg DJ (1997) The surveillance of HIV infection and AIDS in the United Kingdom. Communicable Disease Report, Vol. 7 Review No. 9: 118–20.

Rogers J (1989) Sterilisation in GP surgeries. Nursing Times 85(9): 65–9.

Specification for sharps containers BS7320 (1990)

Appendix 1: Infectious Diseases

Disease	Usual incubation period	Period of communicability	Minimum period of exclusion of patients from school, day nursery, playgroup	Exclusion of family contacts who attend playgroup, day nursery or school
Gastrointestinal illness				
Campylobacter infection	1–10 days 2 days (usually 2–5)	While organism is present in stools, but mainly until diarrhoea is present	Until clinically fit with no diarrhoea for at least 24 hours. Depending on the cause, children attending nursery/playgroup may be excluded for longer periods. Further advice from Consultants in Communicable Control (CCDC). In rare cases, exclusion may be extended and negative stool specimens required. This will be at the discretion of the CCDC	Exclusion not necessary for any contact or family member of the index case. However, if symptoms develop, they should also be excluded until clinically fit with no diarrhoea for at least 24 hours
Cryptosporidiosis	3–11 days (usually 7 days)			
Dysentery	12 hours–7 days (usually 1–3 days)			
Salmonella food poisoning	12–24 hours			
Giardiasis	5–25 days (usually 7–10 days)	While cysts are present in stools, but mainly until diarrhoea is present		
Hepatitis A (infective hepatitis)	2–6 weeks (usually 28–30 days)	From 7–14 days before to 7 days after onset of jaundice	7 days from onset of jaundice and when clinically fit with no symptoms	None
Paratyphoid fever	1–10 days	While organism is present in stools or urine	At the discretion of the CCDC	At the discretion of the CCDC
Typhoid fever	7–21 days (usually 14 days)	While organism is present in stools or urine	At the discretion of the CCDC	At the discretion of the CCDC

Disease	Usual incubation period	Period of communicability	Minimum period of exclusion of patients from school, day nursery, playgroup	Exclusion of family contacts who attend playgroup, day nursery or school
Gastrointestinal illness				
Worms	Variable	Until worms have been treated	Until treated	Family members may require treat-ment
General infections				
Chickenpox	15–18 days	From 1–2 days before and up to 5 days after the appearance of rash	5 days from onset of rash (until spots are dry)	None
Conjunctivitis (viral or bact-erial)	Depends on cause	While symptoms persist	Until treatment has begun and inflammation has started to resolve	None
Fifth disease (slapped cheek syndrome)	6–14 days	Not well known – mainly a few days before appearance of rash	Until clinically well	None
German measles (rubella)	14–21 days	About 7 days before to 4–5 days after onset of rash	5 days from appearance of rash	None
Glandular fever	28–42 days	Prolonged infectious-ness, but once symptoms have subsided, risk is small apart from very close contact, e.g. kissing	Until clinical recovery	None
Hand, foot and mouth disease	3–5 days	Usually while symptoms persist	Until clinically well	None
Measles	10–15 days	A few days before to 4 days after onset of rash	4 days from onset of rash	None
Meningococcal infection (meningitis)	2–10 days (commonly 2–5 days)	While organism is present in nose and mouth	Until clinical recovery. CCDC will advise	No exclusion for contact receiving antibiotic prophylaxis

(contd)

Disease	Usual incubation period	Period of communicability	Minimum period of exclusion of patients from school, day nursery, playgroup	Exclusion of family contacts who attend playgroup, day nursery or school
General infections				
Mumps	12–21 days	From a few days before onset of symptoms to subsidence of swelling (often 10 days)	Until swelling has subsided or when clinically recovered	None
Scarlet fever and other streptococcal infections	1–3 days	While organism is present in the nasopharynx or skin lesion	Until clinical recovery or 48 hours after starting antibiotics	None
Tuberculosis	25–90 days	While organism is present in sputum. Usually non-infectious 2 weeks after starting treatment	CCDC will advise	Screening of contacts is routine policy in cases of pulmonary TB
Whooping cough	10–14 days	7 days after exposure to 21 days after onset of paroxysmal coughing	21 days from onset of paroxysmal coughing	None

Skin infections
Good handwashing is essential if the spread of skin infection is to be reduced. Items such as towels and clothing must not be shared.

Disease	Usual incubation period	Period of communicability	Minimum period of exclusion of patients from school, day nursery, playgroup	Exclusion of family contacts who attend playgroup, day nursery or school
Impetigo (streptococcus pyogenes and staphylococcus aureus)	Usually 4–10 days, but can occur several months after colonization	While lesions remain moist or until 48 hours after starting antibiotic	Until 48 hours after starting antibiotic. Treatment is rapidly effective	None unless they show any signs of infection
Pediculosis capitis (head lice)	Lice eggs hatch in a week and reach maturity in 8–10 days	As long as eggs or lice remain alive	Until after treatment has been undertaken	Examination of family is required and treatment undertaken if necessary

Disease	Usual incubation period	Period of communicability	Minimum period of exclusion of patients from school, day nursery, playgroup	Exclusion of family contacts who attend playgroup, day nursery or school
Skin infections				
Ringworm of the feet (athlete's foot)	Unknown	As long as lesions are present	Exclusion from school or barefoot exercise not necessary once treatment has commenced	None unless they show signs of infection
Ringworm of the scalp	10–14 days	As long as active lesions are present	Exclude until treatment has commenced	None unless they show signs of infection
Ringworm of the body	4–10 days	As long as lesions are present	Exclude until treatment has commenced	None unless they show signs of infection
Scabies	2–6 weeks, but with re-exposure only 1–4 days	Until eggs and mites are destroyed	Exclusion only necessary for 24 hours after treatment	Close contacts, i.e. family, will need treating as they may be incubating scabies.
Verrucae plantaris (plantar warts)	2–3 months, range 1–20 months	Unknown, probably as long as lesion visible	Not necessary. No evidence that wearing of verrucae socks during swimming prevents trans-mission to others	None

CCDC = Consultant in communicable disease control.

Chapter 4
Health promotion

Diana Forster, Diane Pannell and Marilyn Edwards

Health promotion plays a major role in helping to maximize the future health of the nation. Health promotion should be undertaken following an assessment of the needs of a practice population to ensure that strategies are planned appropriately and resources are targeted effectively. The first part of this chapter explains how to assess needs, and examines two less commonly cited areas in which the practice nurse can influence health.

In the second section, pre-conceptual care is discussed. The pre-conception health of both mother and father will influence fertility, the viability of a conception and the outcome of the pregnancy. It is hoped that the issues discussed within this chapter will increase practice nurses' awareness and subsequent pre-conception health advice.

Finally, we shall consider osteoporosis, a major cause of fractures in the elderly, with cost implications for both the individual and the health service. Targeted health promotion can help both in delaying the onset of the disease and in improving compliance in management when the disease is established.

Theories and models of health promotion can be found in excellent health promotion textbooks and are therefore not discussed in this chapter.

Assessing needs

Health needs are changing all the time, so how do we, as nurses, and other health care professionals keep up with the changes and try to meet people's needs effectively? The assessment of health needs has a vital part to play in the current climate of a primary care-led NHS.

One of the key roles of health authorities is to understand how healthy their relevant population is and what its health needs are. As services are prioritized, the limited resources available should be allocated on a basis of need. The provision of health care by interdisciplinary primary health care teams is expanding in scope and importance rather than being seen merely as a gate-keeper to secondary care.

The aim is for people to be able to live at home in their own community, with adequate and relevant health care support when this is needed. In a well-organized general practice, the practice nurse has a key role in assessing the health care needs of the practice population.

A public health approach

General practitioners, practice and community nurses and other health carers increasingly work from a public health as well as a personal health care perspective. This means assessing needs and trends in the health and disease patterns of populations as distinct from individuals.

Health in the new public health-conscious health service, with the first ever Minister for Public Health appointed in 1997, will increasingly be viewed as a personal, family and community responsibility. Epidemiological data from a variety of sources can be put together to provide a picture of health care needs. Demographers seek answers to questions about how many people live in a geographical area, and ascertain age, gender and annual birth, death and marriage figures. Box 4.1 provides definitions of epidemiology and demography.

In order to build a picture of health needs, people who use services should be included when planning, publishing information

---

Box 4.1: Epidemiology and demography (Farmer et al., 1996)

Epidemiology: from the Greek, literally meaning 'studies upon people'. The principal uses of epidemiology have been summarized as:

- the investigation of the causes and natural history of disease, with the aim of disease prevention and health promotion;
- the measurement of health care needs and the evaluation of clinical management, with the aim of improving the effectiveness and efficiency of health care provision

Demography: the study of whole populations of people

and monitoring performance. General practitioner fundholders were required to be accountable to management, patients and the wider public, both financially and professionally. Primary care-led local services should be aware of health needs from a public health perspective, not just reacting to patient demands, but also considering the wider population's needs. For primary health care workers overwhelmed by patient demand, this can be difficult, as illustrated in the Activity 4.1.

Activity 4.1: Consider the following dilemmas (Harris, 1996):

- Should a chronically neurotic woman with a marital problem occupy as much of her general practitioner's time as it would take the general practitioner to carry out annual domiciliary diabetic checks on non-attenders?
- Should mothers with no risk factors receive frequent antenatal checks, which some consider to be of doubtful effectiveness, whilst a Vietnamese community with a high risk of hepatitis A has not received screening or protection?
- Should attenders in a practice be screened opportunistically for diabetes, whilst the majority of the elderly population who may suffer disability from hearing loss are not screened for this, going without adequate hearing assessment and the provision of aids and education?

Client's views

Although incorporating users' views of need into the planning of services has recently received increasing attention, there are methodological difficulties in obtaining service users' views and including them in the policy process. Uncovering needs that cannot be met in practice because of resource constraints also raises ethical issues (Billings and Cowley, 1995).

Difficult choices and policy decisions have to be made when needs are inexhaustible while resources are not. Some examples were presented in the dilemmas in Activity 4.1 above. Similarly, practice nurses often use their knowledge and influence to address the complex needs of homeless people.

A report about tuberculosis and homeless people (Griffiths-Jones, 1997) highlighted the following comprehensive needs:

- reducing the number of homeless people and improving the available accommodation;

- improving nutrition through health education and support;
- the early identification of tuberculosis in homeless people and prompt, successful treatment;
- a thorough contact tracing programme.

The main benefits for homeless clients occur when they receive from practice and community nurses appropriate assessments that identify health and social needs, and are followed up by effective referrals.

Defining health

In order to search for health needs, health itself has to be identified – but health is notoriously difficult to define. It may be defined negatively as the absence of disease, or in a more positive way as a resource for living. The World Health Organization's positive definition embraces a holistic approach (WHO, 1978) including the physical, psychological, emotional and social well-being of a person, group or community.

Health needs therefore encompass education, social services, housing, aspects of the environment and social policy. When estimating health needs, it is important to understand what people themselves mean by 'health'. One research study found that health problems were often played down (Bernard and Meade, 1993). Typically, older women being interviewed would say 'Oh, I'm fine in myself, it's just this ... stiff knee/high blood pressure/trouble with my waterworks....' Health was being assessed by these women not only in terms of the presence or absence of disease, or in terms of functional ability: the women felt well in spite of their illness or disability.

Blaxter (1990) also found in her research that health can be viewed as co-existing with quite severe disease or incapacity. One woman aged 79 and disabled by arthritis said 'To be well in health means I feel I can do others a good turn if they need help.'

Holistic health

Nurses applying a holistic approach to health care place emphasis on the whole person, taking into account each one's physical, emotional, intellectual, spiritual and sociocultural background.

The concept of need in all these aspects of personal care is highly relevant to nursing. When identifying health needs, the focus is upon health promotion, prevention and well-being, helping people to take responsibility for recognizing and meeting their own health needs if possible, and influencing local services and policies.

Nurses need to concentrate on encouraging partnerships between mental health services and local community resources to find ways of meeting people's mental health needs (Repper, 1997).

Defining 'need'

'Need' is a word frequently used in ordinary conversation. In the context of this chapter, however, 'need' becomes a technical term used in a public health framework. Four main types of need in this sense may be identified, based on Bradshaw's (1972) classification:

- *Normative needs*: These are determined or defined by experts or professionals; for example, the components of a healthy diet being explained by a practice nurse based on her expert research into dietetics.
- *Felt needs*: These are identified by patients, users and carers, who, for example, want certain services or treatment to be provided.
- *Expressed needs*: These are needs translated into action, for example by someone visiting a clinic or surgery to seek advice or treatment.
- *Comparative needs*: These are identified by making comparisons between groups, individuals or areas.

Whichever types of need are being considered, it is important that accurate and relevant information is available as a basis for needs assessment at a local or national level. Needs-driven decisions can prevent minority and so-called 'Cinderella' needs being over-looked in favour of patient and professional demands in other areas.

> **Activity 4.2: Identify the main 'Cinderella' sevice needs in the vicinity of your home or workplace. Are there, for example, ethnic minority groups whose needs for advocacy are not being met, elderly, isolated people, single parents, or disabled people needing access to buildings without ramps or lifts?**

Assessing needs for health education

The key to the success of any health teaching activity is identifying the need for it. A practice nurse may identify a need for people with diabetes to learn how to prevent complications by maintaining as near normal blood glucose levels as possible. Teaching patients to balance their diet with insulin or tablets and make adjustments for the effects of exercise, stress and illness would require the practice nurse to be an educator, motivator and supporter in meeting such a need.

Similarly, practice nurses may be involved in setting up advisory sessions for potential travellers, during which health risks abroad, safety in the sun and required vaccination schedules may be discussed, and problems explored.

Decision-maker or victim?

People have more choice and control over some factors affecting their health needs than others. For example, people can choose whether or not to smoke but cannot easily control the atmospheric pollution levels to which they are exposed. Graham (1993), however, discovered in her research that it is not necessarily easy and straight-forward to stop smoking. Mothers in her study reported that smoking was a hard habit to break, although they knew about the health-related problems both for themselves and their children. Living and caring in disadvantaged circumstances, such as inadequate housing and being in debt, meant that smokers clung to the support and comfort provided by their habit, and the women graphically described smoking as a way of coping 'when life's a drag'.

Health care workers have to understand the web of possible influences upon someone's health and well-being in order to assess needs and how to attempt to meet them. For practice nurses, the focus of needs assessment is often at the individual level, but it can also be relevant within the practice and wider community, and at global levels.

WHO and primary health care

Partnerships with clients, patients and the local community form part of the recent movement towards primary health care. Since 'Alma-Ata' (WHO, 1978) the WHO has worked for a shift away from medically dominated, acute-focused services. The key to deliv-

ering 'Health for all by the year 2000' has been identified as primary
health care, linked to improving basic living conditions (Box 4.2).

**Box 4.2: Key principles in the Declaration of Alma-Ata that are vital
for assessing and meeting health needs (WHO, 1978)**

- *Accessibility*: Health care is provided close to where people live and work
- *Acceptability*: Health care is appropriate and provided in ways that people find
  acceptable
- *Equity*: All people have an equal right to health and health care
- *Self-determination*: People have the right and responsibility to make their own
  health choices
- *Community involvement*: People have the right and the responsibility to participate
  individually and collectively in the planning and implementation of their
  health care
- *A focus on health*: Primary health care concentrates on the promotion of health
  as well as on the care of people who are sick, frail or disabled
- *A multisectoral approach*: Housing, food policies, environmental policies and
  social services have an important part to play

The NHS and Community Care Act 1990 and the development
of NHS trust areas throughout the UK has emphasized the change
from service-led to needs-led assessment. Purchasers and commissioners became responsible for contracting services appropriate to
their local population's needs. Nurses were therefore required to
identify the specific needs of patients and patient groups. This
approach requires a variety of changes in the ways in which health
care is shared out and delivered. It depends upon interagency working, health promotion, partnerships with patients and clients, and,
above all, the assessment of health needs.

Practice nurses have a unique part to play in such assessment and
are front-line workers in assessing the health needs of people as individuals and as part of a population group. Primary health care teams
spend much time assessing the needs of individual patients, but less
is usually known about the needs of the practice population. Nurses
need to liaise with other health professionals in making choices
between a vast array of health needs and allocating scarce resources.

The Health of the Nation strategy

An ambitious plan of targets arising out of the theme of 'Health for
all by the year 2000' (WHO, 1978) was published in the Health of
the Nation strategy (DoH, 1992a). Determining priorities and
setting targets were based upon an epidemiological assessment of

health needs. Since then, the scope has broadened, and a new government inquiry was set up to investigate current health needs in the UK.

The initial strategy failed to address issues of poverty in relation to health and issues of food safety, the latter being an area of increasing public health concern. Targets were, however, set in an attempt to meet health needs relating to coronary heart disease and stroke, cancers, mental illness, HIV/AIDS and sexual health, and accidents.

Social class and health needs

One of the founding principles of the NHS was that of equal access to health care according to need for all citizens, regardless of their position in society or where they lived. However, not all social groups have equal access to health care.

Tudor Hart (1971) coined the phrase 'the inverse care law', meaning that health services were generally least available where they were most needed. The greater uptake of preventive and screening services by the non-manual occupations is well documented. Those who actively seek health promotion to meet their health needs are usually those who need it least, and it is far from correct to assume that those who do not turn up for cervical screening do not need it (Victor, 1995).

The widening gap in health inequalities

There are many aspects to equality (Figure 4.1). The 'Variations in Health' report (DoH, 1995) points out that, although mortality rates have fallen steadily, and life expectancy has increased considerably throughout the developed world, there are significant variations in levels of sickness and death between social groups in terms of occupational class, sex, religion and ethnicity, including deaths from preventable diseases.

These differences are increasing in the UK, which underlines the need to reduce inequalities in health. In 1995, although the infant mortality rate for the UK was at its lowest ever, there were still important differences between the social classes.

Deaths were least common for babies whose fathers were in the two highest social classes and were more frequent amongst babies whose fathers were in the lowest (Office for National Statistics, 1997). Poor people have less money to spend on nutritious food, clean water, adequate clothing and shelter, which are all essential to a minimum level of health and well-being.

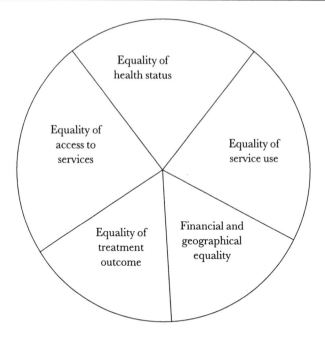

Figure 4.1: Aspects of equality.

Practice and community profiles

Many community nurses have compiled a community profile in the area where they work. Nurses have a valuable part to play in profiling general practitioner practices to assess health and social needs within the practice population (RCN, 1996). Nurses are looking more towards their practice population needs rather than being protective of their own role, and the demarcation lines between practice nurses and other community health nurses are disappearing.

Teamwork is an essential prerequisite for effective health needs assessment. The individual, family, practice and community health profiles kept by health visitors, and increasingly by other community nurses, form a comprehensive database of people's health experience of health care and health needs. The basic principles of health profiling are summarized in Box 4.3.

Box 4.3: Four basic principles of health profiling

- Collecting and analysing information
- Selecting priorities for action
- Choosing nursing activities, including methods of working, for selected priorities
- Evaluating nursing practice

The information collected within a health profile will vary depending upon local circumstances, the type of information (for example, ethnic and age group mix), the culture and the population. However, most should contain information on:

- the incidence of disease, illness, disability and trauma;
- health service provision, such as immunization uptake;
- social and environmental data such as housing, occupation and receipt of welfare benefits (RCN, 1994).

Information for assessing health needs

Victor (1995) distinguishes between three main types of information that may be useful in assessing health needs:

- individual/client-based information;
- data relating to the health status of the community, locality or practice population;
- data concerned with health-related aspects of the community, such as poverty, housing or environment.

The five main issues to be considered when compiling a community profile can be seen in Box 4.4.

Box 4.4: Issues to be considered when compiling a community profile (Billingham, 1994)

- Monitoring and describing the population's health
- Identifying those groups most in need of health support, guidance and treatment
- Identifying the social, economic and environmental factors that have an impact upon people's health
- Taking health action to promote and protect the population's health
- Assessing the impact of health care on health

Gathering data

The age–sex register is one of the most basic pieces of information that is available in every practice. Because the possibility of some conditions occurring depends upon age or gender, such a register can be most useful. Practices vary in the mix of males and females, young and old people, and ethnic groups that they serve. For a comprehensive health needs assessment, however, a wider population than the practice list should be analysed, for example by staging a comparison against national census information. Access to computerized health data facilitates the data collection related to chronic diseases such as cancer and cardiovascular disease.

Office for National Statistics

The Office for National Statistics (ONS) was formed in April 1996 from a merger of the Central Statistical Office and the Office of Population Censuses and Surveys. The ONS aims to bring together all the important data about the lives of everyone in Britain in a way that makes the information accessible.

Independent of any other government department and claiming to be accurate and objective in its reporting of data, the ONS organizes the national system of registering births, deaths and marriages that began in 1837. National, regional and local annual health and population tables are published on separate topics including family statistics, morbidity, population estimates and projections and longitudinal studies. The ONS has the responsibility for the census, which is a major study providing current information that can help to identify health needs and aid future planning.

Census data

Since 1801, there has been a full census every 10 years in Britain, except in 1941 during the Second World War. Data collected are presented by age, marital status, place of residence, occupation of the head of the household, education and many other characteristics that show the changing patterns of populations. In the 1991 census, and for the first time, a question about ethnic origin and country of birth was included. All the information can be broken down into smaller statistical tables, including health authorities, wards and parishes, and is therefore useful in planning health care services and anticipating needs.

Where is such information available?

Local libraries, health promotion and public health departments, and Community Health Councils can be valuable sources of expertise and information, providing publications such as 'Social Trends', 'Population Trends', 'On the State of the Public Health' and the local Director of Public Health's annual report.

Information technology and health profiling

The Public Health Common Data Set is circulated annually to health authorities by the Institute of Public Health. It contains essential information for identifying people at risk and assessing community health needs.

Integrated nursing

Responding to the full range of population health needs is easier to achieve where integrated nursing teams have been developed. The skills, knowledge and experience of a team that includes practice nurses, district nurses, school nurses, community midwives, mental health nurses and health visitors should, for example, enable a wide range of health needs to be identified and prioritized. This would result in an improved health service for the community.

Summary

We have considered many questions that arise in planning health needs assessment, five of the main issues being (Unwin et al., 1997):

- What definition or interpretation of health are we using?
- How do we define a health need?
- What kind of information do we need to make the assessment?
- Where may we find the data that provide the information?
- How do we use the information to make an assessment?

Epidemiological studies are the key to assessing health needs. They can be used to examine local, national and international problems, show changing health trends and disease patterns, and identify groups of people within a community who may be at risk of conditions likely to affect their health and well-being, for example because they are in a particular age group or health category.

Osteoporosis in both men and women, and pre-conceptual care are examples that will be followed up more fully below. Practice nurses are key members of integrated primary health care teams ideally suited to assessing and prioritizing health care needs in the community.

Key points:

1. Need can be normative, felt, expressed or comparative.
2. Needs assessments assure an appropriate allocation of resources.
3. Community profiles are a means of assessing local health care needs.

Promoting pre-conception care

Pre-conception care

Pre-conception care empowers people within the child-bearing range to take responsibility for both their own and their future offspring's health. Preventive care may reduce or eliminate some of the more frequent problems relating to poor nutrition, substance abuse or failure to comply with medical treatment, which may have adverse effects on the conception, pregnancy or perinatal morbidity and mortality rates (Work, 1994).

Preconception screening and interventions are as important as the pregnancy itself in achieving the optimum maternal–fetal outcome (Leuzzi and Scoles, 1996). Ideally, the prospective parents would seek advice from the professionals. This is not always the case for those who actively plan a pregnancy and not an issue for those who become unintentionally pregnant. Health education is of paramount importance for those who seek pre-conception advice. Men also benefit by reassessing their lifestyle and should be included in pre-conception counselling. Preconceptual care by the professional should be seen as a time to educate, screen, diagnose and treat before pregnancy.

Opportunities for pre-conception health education in general practice

Identifying patient needs is an important aspect of the practitioner's role, working within the guidelines of the UKCC's 'Scope of Professional Practice' (1992) and acknowledging professional limitations. The most effective results are seen from a planned package of care with the client. There are many areas in which the lifestyle of either or both prospective parents affects fetal well-being (Figure 4.2) and many opportunities for the nurse to promote pre-conception care (Table 4.1).

Nutrition and maternal weight

The old adage of 'we are what we eat' has a greater importance for the pre-conceptional woman. What she eats not only affects her health, but may also directly influence her ability to conceive or carry a pregnancy to term (Figure 4.2).

Table 4.1: Examples of opportunities to promote pre-conception care within general practice

Well women/men clinics
Family planning clinics
Immunization clinics
Travel vaccination sessions
Pregnancy test results
New patient health checks
Haematological investigations

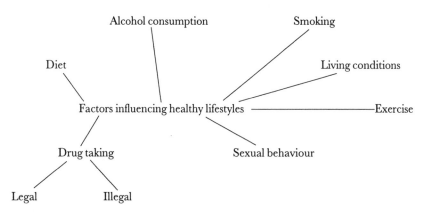

Figure 4.2: Lifestyle factors affecting fetal well-being.

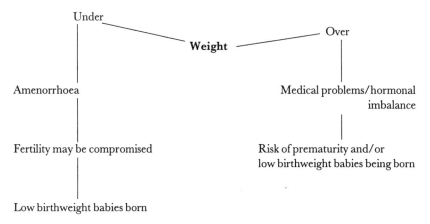

Figure 4.3: Weight and its effects on fertility and fetal well-being.

Women are advised to be within the normal body mass index (BMI) range before commencing pregnancy and are recommended to follow healthy eating guidelines (DoH et al., 1993).

Low BMI has been associated with a reduced ability to conceive and the subsequent pregnancy being at risk. Mothers may deliver low birthweight babies, with all the associated problems, and have an increased risk of sudden infant death syndrome and babies who suffer from respiratory difficulties.

An increased BMI may arise from a medical problem such as polycystic ovary syndrome, in which ovulation is affected and the ability to conceive is reduced. Fertility treatment may be required to correct the hormonal imbalances and improve conception rates. A woman should be encouraged to attain a normal BMI before conception – dieting during pregnancy may result in nutritional imbalance for the mother and fetus. Once disparities in weight have been recognized, steps to rectify the problem by general advice, diet and dietetic consultation should be discussed.

What a woman can and cannot eat during a pregnancy is often perceived as a minefield and is consequently ignored. If appropriate information is provided beforehand, the parents become more familiar with potentially hazardous foods. Whilst some foods should be avoided, the intake of others should be increased. A raised intake of vitamin A (retinoids) has been shown to be teratogenic (DHSS, 1990), and foods with high levels of this vitamin, such as liver and its byproducts, and multivitamin tablets with added vitamin A, are to be avoided. Low levels of zinc have been associated with heart defects and growth retardation. Folic acid, however, has been shown to have beneficial affects on the fetus, reducing the incidence of neural tube defects (see below).

The identification and rebalance of nutritional inadequacies pre-conceptionally will provide a healthier background for both mother and baby.

Folic acid

Folates and folic acid have been conclusively identified as reducing the risk of neural tube defects, such as spina bifida and anencephaly, in developing babies (MRC Vitamin Study Group, 1991). A pre-conceptional increase is of paramount importance as the neural tube (brain and spine) is developed within the first 23–26 days after conception, generally before the woman is aware of a pregnancy. Folates occur naturally in foods (Box 4.5), whereas folic acid is a prepared form of folates.

Women are advised to take folic acid for at least 3 months before conception and for the first 12 weeks of pregnancy (DoH, 1992b). It is recommended that all first-time pregnant women should take 4 µg folic acid daily and increase their dietary folates, giving a total of 6 µg folic acid/folates daily. Women who have had a baby with a neural

---

Box 4.5: Examples of foods containing folates

- *Vegetables*: broccoli, brussel sprouts, cabbage, cauliflower, green beans, peas, potatoes, spinach, sweetcorn, lettuce, tomatoes
- *Most fruits*: bananas, grapefruit, oranges, orange juice
- *Cereals*: brown rice, spaghetti, bread, breakfast cereals fortified with folic acid
- *Other foods*: Marmite, yeast extract, milk (whole or semi-skimmed), yoghurt

---

tube abnormality are advised to take 4 mg folic acid daily and increase their dietary folates. Leaflets and dietary fact-sheets to supplement oral advice should be made readily available in surgery waiting areas, but can be acquired from supermarkets and chemists.

Environmental and lifestyle hazards

Areas that have a great influence on health, and which can be addressed pre-conceptionally, include smoking, alcohol, drugs and infections such as toxoplasmosis.

Smoking

Smoking and its associated health problems are well documented. Less well publicized is the knowledge that smoking can also affect the quality of the sperm and ova; smoking has been shown to cause an increased risk of infertility (Howe et al., 1985). Male fertility is compromised, as sperm from smokers has been found to be decreased in density and motility compared with that of non-smokers (Wynn and Wynn, 1991). This may impede conception.

Impotence is not uncommon, arising from vascular changes reducing the blood flow necessary for an erection. Men may be more inclined to stop smoking if made aware of these vascular changes.

Women who smoke are not only at risk of delayed conception, but also carry an increased risk of early miscarriage (Economides and Braithwaite, 1994). Where a pregnancy is viable, the fetal growth becomes retarded, resulting in stillbirth, premature delivery and/or a low birthweight baby. The babies of parents who smoke are at increased risk of sudden infant death syndrome (Schoendorf and Kiely, 1992).

Alcohol

Alcohol has been shown to affect sperm and ova adversely by affecting the rate of conception and the viability of the conceptus

(Crawley, 1993). One single episode of alcohol abuse around the time of conception has been shown to affect fetal brain growth and increase the risk of congenital malformation. Both parents are advised to avoid alcohol for four months prior to conception.

Although there is no evidence to support fetal abnormalities when one unit of alcohol is consumed by the mother daily, it is still suggested that women avoid alcohol. Women who drink more than six units a day are at risk of their baby developing fetal alcohol syndrome (Ernhart et al., 1987). Heavy drinkers who decrease their alcohol intake pre-conceptionally can reduce the risk of intrauterine growth retardation but not congenital malformation (Day et al., 1989). In these instances, it is essential to work together with the potential parents, and agencies such as Alcoholics Anonymous, to afford the best health care to the parent and baby.

Drugs

Commercially prepared and illegal drugs can affect the developing fetus, particularly during organ development. Consequently, women are advised to avoid the intake of any drug. Women who require medication for medical conditions should seek advice from their doctor. Diabetics require specialist advice.

Illegal drugs are harmful to both mother and fetus, although the extent of this depends largely upon the drugs taken and at what gestation. Heroin usage affects menstruation and ovulation by disrupting the menstrual cycle, although this returns to normal when the heroin is discontinued or replaced with methadone; however, heroin use does not prevent pregnancy (Henderson, 1995).

Anabolic steroid use has been linked with sperm damage, although the effects decrease when the drug is stopped. Sexually active men should be aware that any drug taken may be secreted in their semen and thus greatly affect fetal development (Vallance, 1996).

Potential parents should adopt a drug rehabilitation programme pre-conceptionally and should receive specialist advice from medical sources and the local community drugs team (Institute for the Study of Drug Dependence, 1990).

Infections

Some infections, whilst not causing fertility problems, need to be addressed pre-conceptionally. The sequelae of some infections, such as rubella and toxoplasmosis, can have disastrous effects on both the pregnancy and fetal well-being.

Toxoplasmosis

Although, strictly speaking, toxoplasmosis cannot cause infertility, it can adversely affect pregnancy (Table 4.2). *Toxoplasma gondii* is a microscopic parasite spread predominately through domestic cat faeces and from eating undercooked meats. In the UK, up to half of the population will have toxoplasmosis at some stage during their lives (Toxoplasmosis Trust figures).

The symptoms are similar to those of influenza, so a healthy person may be unaware that he or she has been infected. Diagnosis is by serological screening, performed only by the specialist toxoplasmosis reference laboratories (see below for addresses).

Having entered a human, the parasite can lie dormant, causing no further problems. The infection may be reactivated if the immune system is stressed, for example in pregnant women and those with a depressed immune system. A woman with a first infection of toxoplasmosis is advised to avoid pregnancy for six months.

As the consequences of toxoplasmosis can cause considerable problems for a child, it is important for the practice nurse to address this issue. The incidence of toxoplasmosis infection will be reduced by hygiene advice after handling a cat, ensuring that gloves are worn for gardening, and eating thoroughly cooked meats. Further information on the consequences of toxoplasmosis can be obtained from the Toxoplasmosis Trust (see below for address).

Table 4.2: Effects of toxoplasmosis on pregnancy

Time	Effect
First 3 months	Risk of miscarriage
3rd–6th month	Risk of hydrocephalus and brain lesions causing severe mental retardation and epilepsy
Effects that may not become evident until the child is older	Retinochorditis, which may cause partial-sightedness or blindness

Rubella

Rubella is generally thought of as a childhood infection, although any age group can be at risk. Although rubella does not have any known effects that could prevent conception, problems arise if a woman becomes infected prior to a pregnancy being confirmed. A fetus under 12 weeks' gestation has most risk of developing abnormalities as the infection may interfere with organ development.

The vaccination programme in the UK has ensured that most women, and many younger men, have been vaccinated against rubella infection (DoH, 1996). Despite this programme, 2–5 pregnant women per 100 pregnancies have had neither the infection nor the rubella vaccination (Sense, 1990).

Vaccine-induced antibodies can persist for 18 years, after which the reduced level of immunity may not be adequate to protect a developing fetus against infection (DoH, 1992a). It is advisable for women to have antenatal rubella antibody screening, although pre-conceptional screening is the ideal.

A booster vaccine is offered if the woman has no, or a reduced, rubella immunity. Pregnancy must then be avoided for three months. Vaccine-induced rubella cannot be transmitted to other people but may affect a fetus. A maternal infection does not always mean that the fetus will be affected, and abnormalities will depend on the gestation of the infection (Table 4.3).

Table 4.3: Fetal abnormalities resulting from rubella infection

Stage of gestation	Effect
3–7 weeks gestation	Eye lens develops – cataracts are a typical sign of infection Microphthalmos (uncommon) Pigmentary retinopathy: common but does not affect the sight
6–8 weeks	Heart – structural abnormalities
2–4 months	Ear – hearing problems are common in congenital rubella

Low birthweight babies because the placenta is inefficient

Transient damage – changes in the bones, especially the long bones; purpura, often accompanied by an enlarged liver/spleen; jaundice and inflamed lungs are fairly common side-effects

Sexually transmitted diseases

The contraceptive pill, whilst protecting against conception, does not reduce the risk of sexually transmitted diseases. Cases of acute salpingitis occur exclusively in the sexually active and are due largely to Gonococcus, *Chlamydia trachomatis*, anaerobes, mycoplasmas and Trichomonas.

Chlamydia

Clamydia is an extremely common cause of infertility. A woman may be infected by a partner who has ignored the signs and symptoms of the infection. As chlamydia is usually asymptomatic, the infection may go undetected for many years. Often, the only time the infection, or its antibodies, are detected is when the woman presents to her general practitioner either with pelvic inflammatory disease or because she is unable to conceive.

Early detection and treatment for both partners is preferable. It is often advisable for clients to attend the genito-urinary clinic in their area as the contact tracing of partners is important to avoid further transmission.

Pelvic inflammatory disease causes the Fallopian tubes to become narrowed or completely blocked, requiring surgical intervention.

Syphilis and gonorrhoea

Syphilis and gonorrhoea are also important diseases that require immediate treatment. Undetected and untreated infection may results in transplacental infection of the fetus. A prospective parent who may be at risk from these diseases should be referred to a genito-urinary medicine clinic for screening and treatment.

Genital herpes

Over 90 per cent of women who give birth carry antibodies to herpes simplex virus as a result of past infection. Herpes viruses of the genital area may not affect conception but may result in transplacental infection, leading to fetal death or permanent brain damage.

The incidence of herpes in pregnancy is low in the UK: 13 out of 750 000 babies born annually experience primary infection (Herpes Virus Association, 1995). If the infection is active in the mother at the time of delivery, there is an increased risk of Caesarean section for the birth of the baby, which increases the risk of potential health problems in both the mother and the neonate.

Cytomegalovirus

Cytomegalovirus (CMV), a herpes virus, is one of the most common causes of congenital infection and mental retardation in babies. CMV affects most people, with 90 per cent of infections being asymptomatic and 20–30 per cent of cases occuring in the first year of life. Following a primary infection, the virus can become latent and be reactivated at a later date should the immune system become compromised.

Transmission of this virus can be via body secretions, sexual transmission or transplacental. Maternal infection does not always cause congenital infections, although there is a 25–50 per cent transmission rate during a primary maternal infection to the fetus (Fowler et al., 1992). Unlike the case with rubella infection, there does not appear to be a relationship between gestational age and fetal damage due to CMV.

Positively diagnosed patients should be made aware of the risks of transmission and given appropriate advice, preferably by staff at one of the 200 genito-urinary medicine clinics in England. Referrals may be via a practice nurse or general practitioner, or by self-referral. Women attending specialist clinics can access expert advice, treatment and a confidential contact tracing service.

Readers are recommended to liaise with a local genito-urinary medicine clinic to gain an insight into the management of sexually transmitted diseases.

Teenagers and health care

England and Wales have the highest rate of teenage pregnancy in Western Europe (DoH, 1991). Results from a study of pregnant 16-year-olds in Hull identified the non-use of contraception, living in overcrowded homes and high-density areas, unstable families, smoking at least 10 cigarettes a day and a lack of satisfaction at school as being the common factors found in pregnant teenagers (Konje et al., 1992).

Promoting teenage health through a multidisciplinary approach may reduce the incidence of sexually transmitted disease, cigarette smoking and alcohol abuse in this client group. This may result in an improved pregnancy outcome for girls who become unintentionally pregnant. Liaison with schools and offering support with health issues will help to erode the ignorance that still seems to be apparent across the social strata.

The 'Health of the Nation', document (DoH, 1992a) has identified the need to reduce the rate of conception in under-16-year-olds by at least 50 per cent by the year 2000. Providing good health education to schoolchildren could help towards a healthier future for themselves and any offspring they may one day have.

Genetics

Genetic disorders may result from single gene disorders, chromo-
somal abnormalities or congenital malformations such as neural
tube defects, although many abnormal babies are born to healthy
people with no known risk factors. Between 2 and 3 per cent of
women are at high or recurrent risk of their child having an inherited
disorder (OPCS, 1994).

The House of Commons Health Committee (1991) has acknowledged a need for improved genetic screening. A complete family
medical history will help to identify those at risk of an inherited
disorder. This includes partners who are first cousins or those who
may carry a dominantly inherited genetic defect.

Haemoglobinopathies will identify single gene disorders such as
beta-thalassaemia (Mediterranean origin), sickle cell abnormalities
(Afro-Caribbean origin) and Tay–Sachs Disease (Ashkenazi Jewish
origin). The identification of a disorder, screening for confirmation
and referral for appropriate counselling will provide optimum care
for both parent and baby.

Maternity units will advise on local referral procedures for
genetic counselling.

Role of the practice nurse in pre-conception care

A community profile will highlight specific areas of pre-conceptional
need. These may include data about teenage conceptions that are
not terminated, babies born with neural tube defects, low birthweight babies, drug abusers or the level of sexually transmitted
disease in the locality. Health promotion can then be directed to
meet these needs, supplementing the promotion of healthy lifestyles,
which is an integral part of the practice nurse's role.

There are several areas in which the practice nurse has a key role
in promoting pre-conceptional health (Box 4.6 p. 122). This role
should complement, rather than compete with, advice given by a
midwife or other specialist agency. The practice nurse educates,
facilitates and is a resource for all future parents.

Summary

Pre-conception is the ideal opportunity for a risk assessment of
couples planning a pregnancy. It should also be the time that all men
and women of child-bearing age are given the best health care
advice for themselves and for any future babies, whether planned or

unplanned. It is cost effective to society to reduce the incidence of congenital malformations and infections, with their possible sequelae.

Box 4.6: The practice nurse's role in pre-conception care

- Check rubella status, give vaccine if required and advise the woman to avoid pregnancy for 3 months post-vaccination
- Advise folic acid supplements and increased dietary folates; reinforce the advice with a leaflet
- Advise both prospective parents about the dangers of alcohol and smoking on both fertility and pregnancy
- Exclude chlamydia
- Assess the need for genetic counselling and refer as necessary
- Advise on all aspects of a generally healthy lifestyle

Efficient, effective and appropriate health education can be carried out by the practice nurse in planned and opportunistic consultations. Liaison with other professionals increases the nurses' awareness and knowledge, although they should always be aware of their limitations within their scope of practice. Pre-conception care is the ideal opportunity for prospective parents to attain optimum health for themselves and their future children.

Activity 4.3: Identify one area of pre-conception that you do not currently promote. Discuss with your colleagues how the practice could improve this service.

Key points:

1. Many women have unplanned pregnancies.
2. The health of both prospective parents is important for a healthy baby.
3. The practice nurse is often the first contact for pre-conceptual care.

Osteoporosis

Osteoporosis is a silent disease that is often unrecognized until the sufferer experiences pain from a fracture. It is accepted as a 'female disease' occurring post-menopausally, but it can also affect men and pre-menopausal women, and can be related to many conditions other than simple oestrogen deficiency at menopause. An expert group on osteoporosis has recommended urgent action to halt the increasing incidence of this common disease, which costs Britain an estimated £750 million annually (DoH, 1994).

The disease process of osteoporosis will be examined in order to enable the reader to identify areas in which health promotion may be appropriate in his or her working environment. This is essential in order to maximize bone density for vulnerable groups and delay the onset of this condition. Emphasis is placed on practical nursing interventions; medical management will be mentioned only where appropriate.

Definition

Osteoporosis is a reduction in bone density that is sufficient to compromise the skeleton so that a fracture may occur after minimal trauma.

Bone formation

The formation, resorption and repair of bone are controlled by several hormones (Figure 4.4). The maximum growth spurt for girls is at 11–15 years of age, slightly later than that for boys (National Osteoporosis Society, 1989), whilst peak bone mass is usually achieved by the age of 30 (Peel and Eastell, 1996).

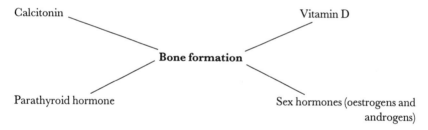

Calcitonin stops osteoclasts dissolving bone when there is a high calcium level in the blood. *Vitamin D* increases calcium absorption from food in the gut and plays an important part in bone formation. *Parathyroid hormone* maintains the level of calcium in the blood and also acts on the kidneys, reducing the loss of calcium in the urine and increasing the absorption of calcium from food in the gut. The *sex hormones* allow bone cells to respond fully to the other major controlling hormones.

Figure 4.4: Hormone influences on bone formation (Dixon and Woolf, 1989).

Human bone is continually being resorbed and reformed, about 10 per cent of the adult skeleton being remodelled each year (Peel and Eastell, 1996); bone loss results from an imbalance between resorption and formation. After skeletal maturity, bone is lost in both sexes at about 1 per cent a year, although women have an accelerated bone loss for 5–10 years post-menopause. However, some elderly people show no signs of bone loss (Swedish Council on Technology Assessment in Health Care, 1997).

Epidemiology

One in four (22%) women over 50 years of age in Britain have low bone density, which predisposes them to osteoporotic fractures (National Dairy Council, 1996), one in three women and one in 12 men suffering from an osteoporotic fracture at some time in their lives (Selby, 1997). There is a 10–20 per cent mortality over the subsequent six months following a hip fracture, whilst 50 per cent of sufferers will be unable to walk without help and 25 per cent will require long-term domiciliary care (Riggs and Melton, 1995).

Classification of osteoporosis

- *Post-menopausal osteoporosis* results from accelerated bone loss, probably as a result of oestrogen deficiency. Typically, women in their 60s and 70s present with distal forearm fractures and crushed lumbar or thoracic vertebra. The latter is the most common osteoporotic fracture, 25 per cent of women having evidence of this by the age of 75 years (Whitehead and Godfrey, 1992). Other less common sites are the humerus, ribs and pelvis.
- *Senile osteoporosis* results from the slower age-related bone loss that occurs in men and women, typically manifesting at the femoral neck.
- *Secondary osteoporosis* is related to other diseases (Box 4.7) and accounts for about 20 per cent of cases in women and 40 per cent in men.

Box 4.7: Secondary diseases as causes of osteoporosis (Dennison and Cooper, 1996; Peel and Eastell, 1996; Cohen et al., 1997; Rosen, 1997)

- Hyperthyroidism*
- Diabetes*
- Malabsorption
- Chronic liver disease
- Ischaemic heart disease
- Systemic lupus erythematosus
- Epilepsy**
- Rheumatoid arthritis
- Myeloma

*The correction of hypo- or hyperfunction of an endocrine gland can increase bone mineral density
**Medication can adversely affect bone metabolism

Risk factors

The two main factors that determine whether or not a woman will develop osteoporosis are the peak pre-menopausal adult bone mass and the rate of post-menopausal bone loss. The main risk factors are listed in Table 4.4, and the protective factors in Box 4.8.

Endocrine disorders are the most frequent cause of secondary osteoporosis in men and women, whilst the risk to patients on long-term corticosteroids, including those with rheumatoid arthritis, brittle asthma and systemic lupus erythematosus, cannot be overestimated.

McGee (1997) discusses the association between intramuscular contraception that leads to secondary amenorrhoea and the risk of osteoporosis; young amenorrhoeic women may lose as much as 2–6 per cent of their bone mass each year.

Table 4.4: Risk factors for osteoporosis

Factor	Rationale
Being female	1 in 3 women will suffer an osteoporotic fracture at some time in their lives
Being a smoker	May lead to early menopause and oestrogen deficiency
High alcohol consumption	Suppresses bone formation and may lead to hypogonadism
Prolonged inactivity/ immobility	Weight-bearing exercise stengthens bone
Thin frame	May fail to achieve peak bone mass
Heredity	Genetic factors may account for up to 70% of the variability in peak bone mass
Hypogonadism	Androgens are necessary for bone formation
Race	Being white or oriental increases the risk
Corticosteroids	Those on long-term oral steroids (7.5 mg per day), e.g. for brittle asthma
Oestrogen deficiency amenorrhoea	Of more than 6 months. May be due to natural causes or to underweight, anorexia, excessive exercise or treatment for endometriosis
Being elderly	An accelerated rate of bone loss occurs following the menopause, 50% of a woman's bone mass being lost by the age of 75 years
Premature menopause or hysterectomy before the menopause	Under 40 years of age

Data from: Stevenson, 1995; Dennison and Cooper, 1996; Peel and Eastell, 1996; Rosen, 1997; RCN, 1997; Segal and Lane, 1997.

Box 4.8: Factors protecting against osteoporosis (Dixon and Woolf, 1989)

- Early menarche, before the age of 13
- Late menopause, after the age of 55
- Having had several children
- Breastfeeding
- Taking the oral contraceptive pill
- Being a non-smoker
- Being overweight
- Being active from childhood
- Being well nourished as a child, with a high calcium intake

Activity 4.4: Referring to Table 4.4, identify your practice population that is 'at risk' of osteoporosis. Consider local demography, including age and socio-economic distribution, and secondary factors.

Identification of at-risk patients

People at risk of osteoporosis may be identified through a disease register or computer analysis of diagnosis and/or medication. Routine height checks give only a rough estimate of possible risk and have limited value in establishing the level of bone density in an individual (Swedish Council of Technology Assessment in Health Care, 1997) but may identify people with height loss who should be referred for further assessment. It may be useful to devise a protocol for practice use in order to ensure that all the doctors and nurses are using the same criteria. Nurses must also be alert for young women with secondary amenorrhoea, whatever the cause.

There are few investigations to diagnose osteoporosis, and in many cases no investigations are undertaken at all until the patient complains of pain or has experienced a hip or wrist fracture.

Straight X-rays

A spinal X-ray will identify existing fractures, although a straight X-ray can detect osteoporosis only when 30 per cent of the bone mass is lost. It is highly likely that when osteoporosis is detected through straight X-ray examination the sufferer will already have experienced pain or had an injury giving rise to a fracture as a result of osteoporosis.

Bone densiometry

Bone densiometry is usually measured by dual X-ray absorptiometry (DEXA scanning). This technique uses low-dose radiation to measure accurately bone mineral density, usually of the lumbar spine and proximal femur. Some methods measure the forearm or heel bone, while others measure several sites simultaneously.

This is a reliable method of predicting a person's risk of fracture. It can also be used to monitor the response to treatment. Unfortunately, access to scanners may in some areas be limited because of a lack of awareness and/or cost implications. In some health authorities, these services are available to women who are prepared to pay, although those women most at risk of osteoporosis may be those least able to pay.

Management of established osteoporosis

The goals of treatment for patients with established osteoporosis are to:

- maintain normal bone;
- prevent the deterioration of normal bone to osteoporotic bone.

Secondary causes

The monitoring and correction of an underlying secondary cause, such as hypo- or hyperfunction of endocrine glands, giving rise to, for example, thyroid disorders and diabetes, can increase bone mineral density (Rosen, 1997). A simple audit and protocol could redress any deficiencies in current management (see Chapter 2).

Medication

Drugs used to treat established osteoporosis prevent further bone loss and and can reduce the risk of further fractures by up to 50 per cent (Peel and Eastell, 1996) (Box 4.9).

Prevention of osteoporosis through health promotion

Although the terms 'health promotion' and 'health education' are often used interchangeably, McKnight and Edwards (1998) make the point that health promotion can appear coercive and aggressive instead of merely educative. You may wish to bear this in mind when planning any health promotion activities.

Box 4.9: Medication to treat established osteoporosis

- Hormone replacement therapy, which has an anti-resorptive factor reducing bone loss but does not increase bone density
- Anabolic steroids may have been more popular before the advent of newer therapies, but the androgenic side-effects (especially the growth of facial hair) have made them unacceptable for most women
- Calcium and vitamin D supplements are reported to be useful in elderly patients but are probably ineffective in peri-menopausal women (Peel and Eastell, 1996)
- Calcitonin is an anti-resorptive hormone, usually given with calcium and vitamin D, to prevent bone loss; it may lead to an increase in bone density
- Biphosphonates reduce osteoclastic activity (the breakdown of bone) and increase vertebral bone mineral density. This then lowers the risk of vertebral crush fractures

---

Most of the data on osteoporosis involve post-menopausal women as they are the largest group at risk of this disease. It has been noted above, however, that there are a range of at-risk groups for which health education and health promotion is essential.

The importance of diet in young women has received a higher profile during the late 1990s with recognition that calcium intake in this group is unacceptably low and incompatible with maximizing peak bone mass (see Chapter 7). An update by the National Dairy Council highlighted calcium intake to be inversely related to social class, with lone mothers having a significantly lower dietary calcium level (National Dairy Council, 1996). Slimmers also have a tendency to reduce their dairy, and therefore calcium, intake, which compromises their skeletal health. This suggests that health promotion must focus not on middle-aged and elderly women (recognized 'women at risk') but on the whole female population.

Lifestyle advice is a key area in primary health care and is incorporated, in part, in most health interventions. It may be necessary to review current policy to ensure that appropriate health promotion is offered to a wider population in order to delay the onset of osteoporosis.

The author has assumed that readers already undertake health promotion using poster displays, leaflets, one-to-one counselling and groupwork. Other methods, such as community initiatives, are more difficult to organize and require the commitment of several health disciplines or associated agencies. However, these initiatives are challenging, target a wider audience and can be worth the effort.

The different models of health promotion will not be discussed, but their theories are implicitly incorporated into general health care, which will relate to primary, secondary and tertiary prevention (Naidoo and Wills, 1994). In the context of osteoporosis, these are as follows:

- *Primary prevention* (A) aims to prevent the onset of osteoporosis and may relate to all age groups.
- *Secondary prevention* (B) involves alleviating pain and reducing further fractures once osteoporosis is established.
- *Tertiary prevention* (C) refers to assisting people with chronic or irreversible ill-health to cope with their condition and maximize their health potential. Multiple osteoporotic vertebral crush fractures lead to severe kyphosis, which is irreversible.

Health promotion for each of the three stages of health prevention overlaps – these stages being, for convenience, referred to as A, B and C in the following text.

Children and young women

There have been several studies that support the influence of diet and exercise at the time of pubertal growth (National Dairy Council, 1996; Selby, 1997). Smoking, excess alcohol consumption and excess salt intake (from salty snacks and processed foods) are all detrimental to the skeleton but are commonly a daily part of the teenage lifestyle.

One health promotion strategy to maximize peak bone mass in girls involved a multidisciplinary approach (Figure 4.5 p. 130) (Edwards, 1997). Although the girls did not appear to increase their dietary calcium intake, the campaign reached other vulnerable groups and raised the general awareness of diet and physical activity related to bone health. Simple areas to address include walking to school when possible and substituting milk for sugary drinks.

Unfortunately, teenagers are often unreceptive to health promotion, so health promotion (A) must target children and their parents to achieve maximum peak bone mass to promote strong bones that will last a lifetime.

Vegans

Vegan diets are often high in roughage, which may hinder calcium absorption from other foods. This is also relevant when people are encouraged to eat a low-fat, high-fibre diet. It is essential to assess any diet for adequate calcium intake as calcium supplements may sometimes be necessary (A, B, C). A dietitian will usually be willing to offer advice.

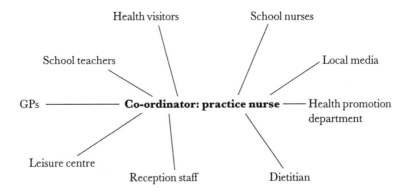

Figure 4.5: Multidisciplinary approach to health promotion.

Exercise

Regular physical activity has a beneficial effect on the skeleton and should be encouraged from an early age (A). Bone is strengthened through weight-bearing exercises such as walking, dancing and aerobics, although excessive exercise can have an adverse effect on bone growth. Other benefits of exercise include improved balance, which reduces accidents and falls (B, C), and improved general well-being.

Health promotion must be targeted to need. In areas with low car ownership, children may well take plenty of exercise, so the emphasis will lie on other areas of health.

Alcohol

Alcohol damages bone cells and reduces calcium absorption. From the author's observations, people who drink excessively often smoke, eat a diet low in calcium and take limited exercise. Health promotion should include advice on alcohol consumption, and support, for women of all ages (A, B, C).

Post-menopausal women

Hormone replacement therapy

It has been reported that premature menopause affects 1 per cent of all women under the age of 40 years (RCN, 1997). Hormone replacement therapy (HRT) is the most effective preventive measure against osteoporosis (A); oestrogen treatment given for 10 years post-menopause is reported to delay the onset of osteoporosis for 10 years and delay the expected peak of femoral fractures until close to the expected span of life (Coope, 1993). Dennison and Cooper (1996) quote studies concluding that this time limit is controversial and unsatisfactory.

Most women do not want to take hormones (Coope, 1993), but they do need education about the possible benefits of HRT and other lifestyle factors that affect their future health. This advice needs to be offered at the time when it is most effective – just before or just after the menopause. Nurses have the knowledge and resources to offer unbiased information, which, when supported by literature, can allow women to make an informed choice about their health.

HRT has been shown to be an effective first-line therapy for established osteoporosis (B) (RCN, 1997).

Compliance with treatment (A, B, C)

Between 20 and 30 per cent of women stop HRT within six months. Gupta and Kenney (1997) offer advice on how to encourage compliance with HRT (Box 4.10), which can be adapted to any treatment. Nurses have a key role in encouraging compliance with treatment or suggesting an alternative method of treatment delivery. Regular follow-ups with the nurse allows the woman to discuss any concerns, may lead to improved levels of compliance and offers opportunities to discuss any other related health issues such as diet, smoking cessation and exercise.

Box 4.10: How to encourage compliance with hormone replacement therapy (adapted from Gupta and Kenney, 1997)

This approach utilizes the expertise and knowledge of each discipline and improves overall awareness within the community

- Detailed counselling on first visit – offer supportive literature, videos or tapes. Consider the language needs of ethnic minorities
- Education on minor side-effects (see point above).
- Regular follow-ups – allows continuing support
- Telephone helplines at specialist menopause clinics are popular and useful
- May prefer an alternative method – refer to GP

Maintaining bone strength

It is essential to maintain any remaining bone through dietary calcium and vitamin D synthesis (B, C). Eating small, frequent meals will reduce discomfort from the abdominal distension that often accompanies kyphosis.

The recommended daily calcium intake for women aged 50–65 years is 1500 mg if not on HRT, and 1000 mg if taking HRT (National Dairy Council, 1996). This information can be promoted through simple dietary advice during any consultation.

Weight-bearing exercise should also be encouraged. People with spinal osteoporosis (B, C) are encouraged to exercise to improve posture, balance and breathing (Dixon and Woolf, 1989). A physiotherapist may be willing to offer advice for a specific client.

Accident prevention

The risk of falls increases with alcohol consumption, whilst an increased risk of falls in epileptic patients can be related to drug toxicity (Cohen et al., 1997). Drug regimes in these patients, and for those for whom multiple drugs are prescribed, may need reviewing by the doctor. Patients with a visual impairment should be referred to an optician for advice in order to reduce the risk of falls.

Analgesia

Long-term analgesia may be required to control the pain in established osteoporosis (B, C). Exercises to improve posture may alleviate some pain, while referral to a physiotherapist for alternative methods of pain relief, for example electrical stimulation (TENS), may be helpful.

Osteoporosis in men

Osteoporotic fractures in men occur most commonly at the hip, usually as a result of some other condition or treatment, for example corticosteroids, although hypogonadism is reported to be a major risk factor for osteoporosis in men (Hahn, 1993). An increase in bone formation and a decrease in resorption can be achieved with testosterone treatment. Nurses may be involved in treatment compliance and offering support for these men. Although many of the treatments used in women are likely to be effective in men, there is no licensed treatment for osteoporosis in men. Men should therefore be referred for specialist assessment and treatment (Selby, 1997).

> **Activity 4.5: Devise a health promotion strategy to maintain bone strength for men and women with established osteoporosis.**

Summary

As demography changes with increased longevity, the morbidity and mortality of osteoporosis are also set to increase. Although everyone loses bone through ageing, only some will suffer the consequences until very elderly. Nurses must use their excellent communication skills to identify people at risk of osteoporosis and promote the benefits of a healthy lifestyle to reduce the premature loss of bone.

Women who would benefit from oestrogen therapy to protect their bones must be offered as much support as they require to ensure that they continue therapy for the recommended length of time. They must have access to relevant and unbiased information about HRT and its alternatives, which should be supported with information literature, videos and books as required. Provision may need to be made for women with language difficulties and special needs.

Men's health needs with respect to bone conservation are currently neglected, although this area may be addressed in the future. Holistic care for all people will include this client group in general health promotion initiatives.

In the new primary care-led NHS, the National Health Service Executive has required commissioners to 'improve the cost effectiveness of services throughout the NHS, and thereby secure the greatest health gain from the resources available' (Health Education Authority, 1997). Although the cost-effectiveness of primary health prevention in reducing or delaying osteoporosis cannot be measured for many years, nurses themselves have the resources to promote strong bones from the cradle to the grave.

Key points:

1. Osteoporosis affects men and women of all age groups.
2. Effective health promotion can delay the onset of the disease.
3. Health promotion can improve compliance with the management of established disease.

References

Bernard M, Meade K (1993) Women Come of Age. London: Edward Arnold.

Billingham K (1994) Beyond the individual. Health Visitor 67(9): 295.

Billings JR, Cowley S (1995) Approaches to community needs assessment: a literature review. Journal of Advanced Nursing 22: 721–30.

Blaxter M (1990) Health and Lifestyles. London: Tavistock/Routledge.

Bradshaw JS (1972) A taxonomy of social need. In McLachlan G (Ed.) Problems and Progress in Medical Care: Essays on Current Research, 7th series. London: Oxford University Press.

Cohen A, Lancman M, Mogul H, Marks S, Smith K (1997) Strategies to protect bone mass in the older patient with epilepsy. Geriatrics 52(8): 70–81.

Coope J (1993) Menopause. In Macpherson A (Ed.) Women's problems in General Practice. Oxford: Oxford University Press.

Crawley H (1993) Plan before conception for a healthy pregnancy. MIMS 19 January: 24–9.

Day NL, Jasperse D, Richardson G (1989) Prenatal exposure to alcohol: effect on infant growth and morphological characteristics. Paediatrics 84: 536–41.

Dennison E, Cooper C (1996) The epidemiology of osteoporosis. British Journal of Clinical Practice 50(1):33–6.

Department of Health (1991) On the State of Public Health. London: HMSO.

Department of Health (1992a) The Health of the Nation: A Strategy for Health in England. Cm 1986. London: HMSO.

Department of Health (1992b) Folic Acid and the Prevention of Neural Tube Defects. Report from an Expert Advisory Group. London: HMSO.

Department of Health (1994) Advisory Group on Osteoporosis Report. London: DoH.

Department of Health (1995) Variations in Health. London: HMSO.

Department of Health (1996) Immunisation Against Infectious Diseases. London: HMSO.

Department of Health and Social Security (1990) Vitamin A and Pregnancy. Letter from the Chief Medical and Nursing Officers DL/CMO(90)11, PL/CNO(90)10. London: DoH.

Department of Health, General Medical Services Committee, Royal College of General Practitioners (1993) Better Living, Better Life (special working edition). Henley-on-Thames: Knowledge House.

Dixon A, Woolf A (1989) Avoiding Osteoporosis. London: Macdonald.

Economides D, Braithwaite J (1994) Smoking, pregnancy and the fetus. Journal of the Royal Society of Health 114: 198–201.

Edwards M (1997) A Strategy to Maximise Peak Bone Mass. 1996 NDC/RCGP Practice Team Nutrition Award. Unpublished document.

Ernhart CB, Sokol RJ, Martier S et al. (1987) Alcohol teratogenicity in the human: a detailed assessment of specificity, critical period, and threshold. American Journal of Obstetrics and Gynecology 156: 33–9.

Farmer R, Miller D, Lawrenson R (1996) Lecture Notes on Epidemiology and Public Health Medicine, 4th Edn. Oxford: Blackwell Science.

Fowler KB, Stagno PHS, Pass RF, Britt WJ, Boll TJ, Alford CA (1992) The outcome of congenital cytomegalovirus infection in relation to maternal antibody status. New England Journal of Medicine 325: 663–7.

Graham H (1993) When Life's a Drag: Women, Smoking and Disadvantage. London: HMSO.

Griffiths-Jones A (1997) Tuberculosis in homeless people. Nursing Times 93(9): 60–1.

Gupta S, Kenney A (1997) The menopause and HRT. Update 55(5): 304–14.

Hahn TJ (1993) Metabolic bone disease. In Kelley WN, Harris ED, Ruddy S, Sledge CB (Eds) Textbook of Rheumatology. Philadelphia: WB Saunders.

Harris A (1996) What is a primary care-led policy? In Littlejohns P, Victor C (Eds) Making Sense of a Primary Care-led Health Service. Oxford: Radcliffe Medical Press.

Health Education Authority (1997) Achieving Health Gain through Health Promotion in a Primary Care-led NHS. London: HEA.

Henderson S (1995) Drug Information for Women: Drugs and your Health. London: Institute for the Study of Drug Dependence.

Herpes Virus Association (1995) Herpes Simplex: A Guide. London: Wilton Wright & Son.

House of Commons Health Committee (1991) Maternity Services: Preconception. The Fourth Report. London: HMSO.

Howe G, Westoff C, Vessey M, Yeates D (1985) Effects of age, cigarette smoking and other factors on fertility; findings of a large prospective study. British Medical Journal 290: 1967.

Institute for the Study of Drug Dependence (ISSD) (1990) Drugs, Pregnancy and Childcare – A Guide for Professionals. London: ISSD.

Konje JC, Palmer A, Watson A, Hay DM, Imrie A, Ewings P (1992) Early teenage pregnancies in Hull. British Journal of Obstetrics and Gynaecology 99: 969–73.

Leuzzi RA, Scoles KS (1996) Preconception counselling for the primary care physician. Medical Clinics of North America 80(2): 337–74.

McGee C (1997) Secondary amenorrhoea leading to osteoporosis: incidence and prevention. Nurse Practitioner 22(5): 38–63.

McKnight S, Edwards M (1998) Health promotion. In Blackie C (Ed.) Community Health Care Nursing. Edinburgh: Churchill Livingstone.

MRC Vitamin Study Group (1991) Prevention of neural tube defects: results of the Medical Research Council Vitamin Study. Lancet 238: 131–7.

Naidoo J, Wills J (1994) Health Promotion: Foundations for Practice. London: Baillière Tindall.

National Dairy Council (1996) Calcium and Bone Health Topical Update No. 7. London: NDC.

National Osteoporosis Society (1989) Calcium. Recommended Daily Allowances. London: NOS.

Office for National Statistics (1997) Social Trends 27. London: Stationery Office.

Office of Population Censuses and Surveys (1994) Congenital Malformations Statistics: Notifications 1992. Series MB3(8). London: HMSO.

Peel N, Eastell R (1996) Osteoporosis. In Snaith M (Ed.) ABC of Rheumatology. London: BMJ Publishing Group.

Repper J (1997) Fear and loathing. Nursing Times 93(29): 42–4.

Riggs BL, Melton LJ (1995) The worldwide problem of osteoporosis: insights afforded by epidemiology. Bone 17(5, supplement): 505S–511S.

Rosen CJ (1997) Endocrine disorders and osteoporosis. Current Opinion in Rheumatology 9(4): 355–61.

Royal College of Nursing (1994) Public Health: Nursing Rises to the Challenge. London: RCN.

Royal College of Nursing (1996) Profiling Poverty: A Guide for Nurses in the Community. London: RCN.

Royal College of Nursing (1997) The Menopause, Hormone Replacement Therapy and Osteoporosis. London: RCN.

Schoendorf KC, Kiely JL (1992) Relationship of sudden infant death syndrome to maternal smoking during and after pregnancy. Paediatrics 90: 905–8.

Segal LG, Lane NE (1997) Osteoporosis and systemic lupus erythematosus: etiology and treatment strategies. Annales de Médécine Interne 147(4): 281–9.

Selby PL (1997) Osteoporosis. Update 54(4): 228–36.

Sense (1990) Rubella in pregnancy. What does it do? London: 1.

Stevenson JC (1995) The impact of bone loss in women with endometriosis. International Journal of Gynaecology and Obstetrics 50 (supplement 1): S11–S15.

Swedish Council on Technology Assessment in Health Care (1997) Bone density measurement – a systematic review. A review from SBU, the Swedish Council on Technology Assessment in Health Care. Journal of Internal Medicine 739 (supplement): 1–60.

Tudor Hart J (1971) The inverse care law. Lancet 1: 405–12.

United Kingdom Central Council for Nursing, Midwifery and Health Visiting (1992) Scope of Professional Practice. London: UKCC.

Unwin N, Carr S, Leeson J, Pless-Mulloli T (1997) An Introductory Study Guide to Public Health and Epidemiology. Buckingham: Open University Press.

Vallance P (1996) Drugs and the fetus. British Medical Journal 312: 1053–4.

Victor C (1995) Information and health promotion. In Pike S, Forster D (Eds) Health Promotion for all. Edinburgh: Churchill Livingstone.

Whitehead M, Godfrey V (1992) Hormone Replacement Therapy. Edinburgh: Churchill Livingstone.

Work BA (1994) Screening general obstetric populations for risk assessment. Who will need testing? Clinics in Perinatology 21(4): 699–705.

World Health Organization (1978) Primary Health Care: Report of the International Conference on Primary Health Care, Alma-Ata, USSR, 6–12 September 1978. Geneva: WHO.

Wynn M, Wynn A (1991) The Case for Preconception Care of Men and Women. Oxford: AB Academic Publishers.

Further reading

Billings JR (1996) Assessing health needs. In Twinn S, Roberts B, Andrews S (Eds) Community Health Care Nursing: Principles for Practice. Oxford: Butterworth-Heinemann.

Dixon A, Woolf A (1989) Avoiding Osteoporosis. London: Macdonald.

Hahn TJ (1993) Metabolic bone disease. In Kelley WN, Harris ED, Ruddy S, Sledge CB (Eds) Textbook of Rheumatology. Philadelphia: WB Saunders.

McGee C (1997) Secondary amenorrhoea leading to osteoporosis: incidence and prevention. Nurse Practitioner 22(5): 38–63.

McKnight S, Edwards M (1998) Health promotion. In Blackie C (Ed.) Community
    Health Care Nursing. Edinburgh: Churchill Livingstone.
Naidoo J, Wills J (1994) Health Promotion: Foundations for Practice. London:
    Baillière Tindall.
Wilkinson R (1996) Unhealthy Societies: The Afflictions of Inequality. London:
    Routledge.

Useful addresses

The Amarant Trust,
11–13 Charterhouse Buildings,
London EC1M 7AN
Tel: (01891) 660620
Provides information about menopause-related issues.

The National Osteoporosis Society,
PO Box 10,
Radstock,
Bath BA3 3YB
Tel: (01761) 471771   Helpline: (01761) 472721

The Toxoplasmosis Trust,
61 Collier Street,
London N1 9BE
Tel: 0171–713 0663   Helpline: 0171–713 0599

Sense (The National Deaf, Blind and Rubella Association)
11–13 Clifton Terrace,
London N4 3SR
Tel: 0171–272 7774

The Sickle Cell Society,
54 Station Road,
London NW10 4UA
Tel: 0181–961 7795/4006

Toxoplasmosis Reference Laboratories:

St George's Hospital,
Blackshaw Road,
London SW17 0QT

Singleton Hospital,
Sgeti,
Swansea,
Dyfed SA2 8QA

Raigmore Hospital,
Inverness IV2 3UJ

Chapter 5
Men's health

Marilyn Edwards, Glenn Turp and Jean Crutchley

Any audit of general practice consultations will confirm that men attend less frequently than women. Mortality figures show that, although both sexes are living longer, men still on average die younger than women. This chapter examines the social issues surrounding men's health and tries to identify why men are often reluctant to seek medical advice or accept health education.

There is an assumption that all men are heterosexual unless they state otherwise. The key issues relating to the health of men who have sex with men are explored in the second part of this chapter through the male author's experience of working with men and through his own experience. The underlying problems may challenge the reader's current thinking about this topic.

Testicular and prostate cancer have been included in this chapter to highlight the nurse's role in promoting health and encouraging men to seek medical advice at an early stage of a disease process. Although the early detection and treatment of malignancy reduce mortality from testicular cancer, the benefits of prostate screening are controversial. The reader will, however, have access to the facts to share with men who want information about these diseases.

Social issues surrounding men's health

Men are physically more vulnerable than women from the moment they are conceived until they die (Nicholson, 1993). Although their health needs are apparently greater than those of women, these appear to be inadequately addresssed. The importance of men's health, and the scope for men to improve their health, has been recognized by the Department of Health (DoH, 1993), although Lloyd (1996) highlights current issues for concern that centre on the lack of a definition of men's health.

Issues relating to inequalities of health are paramount to men's health; those specific to homosexuality are covered in the following section of this chapter.

Gender

The higher male mortality may be attributed to physiological sex differences, including a slightly higher risk of birth injury and asphyxia resulting from male babies being on average slightly larger than females, and a higher rate of genetically transmitted disorders (Morgan et al., 1985). Mortality rates for men have remained markedly higher than for females. The predicted life expectancies for boys and girls born in Britain in 1985 is 72 years and 78 years respectively (Bone et al., 1995).

Health

Health is a complex issue influenced by the social, economic, cultural and physical environment in which people live.

Health has been defined negatively as the absence of disease, functionally as the ability to cope with everyday activities, and positively as fitness and well-being (Blaxter, 1990). Definitions of health and illness vary between cultures, subcultures and communities.

Health and masculinity

The foundations of masculinity are laid down in boyhood, when boys are socialized into acceptable masculine behaviour. Men are encouraged to 'make the best of a bad job', develop a 'stiff upper lip', be self-reliant and tolerate pain.

Socialization is continued through the media, where men are portrayed as heroes and workers, able to cope with everyday stress and to solve their own problems. The male gender role stereotype demands 'real' men to be healthy, strong and self-sufficient.

Masculine competitive and aggressive characteristics may also predispose men to certain stress-related health problems. A competitive, striving personality trait (type A) is associated with an increased risk of coronary heart disease (Nicholson, 1993).

The monotony of work and the fear of unemployment, housing problems, poverty and family crises were identified as stressors over a decade ago (Morgan et al., 1985); there is no reason to believe that these stressors are any less significant now.

Married men tend to be healthier and have better jobs than do single men of all ages (Nicholson, 1993). Although there appear to be no data on this issue, men co-habiting with a partner of either sex may be included in this category. Risks of premature death from all causes are closely related to marital status, and the loss of a partner through death, separation or divorce poses important threats to health.

Men in Western societies are brought up to value work as an end in itself and to fix their identities around particular occupations, where friendship and financial reward may compensate for the threat of redundancy.

Alcohol may be a support for men who are reluctant to express their emotional and personal needs or to seek support from each other (Nicholson, 1993).

Men's health and social class

Much of the documentation on gender and health relates to the inequalities of health resulting from social class. Major differences exist in all aspects of health, with a gradual deterioration from class I to class IV and a marked deterioration in social class V (Townsend et al., 1992). Health affects social mobility: ill-health can result in a drop in social class.

The most important factor that determines the way in which a person deals with a symptom appears to be his or her internal belief structure about the meaning of symptoms and illness. Health is considered a good quality, and few respondents of one study wanted to say that they were anything but healthy (Morgan et al., 1985). Illness is perceived as a state of spiritual or moral malaise. Lower social groups consider only serious conditions as illness.

It has been argued that the diseases causing premature death, in particular heart disease and cancer, are closely linked with male lifestyle in our society (Armstrong, 1994).

Coronary heart disease (CHD) accounts for 29 per cent of all male deaths, men in social class V being nearly three times more likely to die prematurely from CHD than men in social class I (HEA, 1990).

Alcohol consumption and the level of cigarette smoking are reported to increase with declining class, especially amongst men (Townsend et al., 1992). This is not supported by an epidemiological study by the DoH (1996a) concluding that there is little difference between the proportions of employed and unemployed men who drink more than the recommended level of 21 units a week.

Men's health and employment

Men are stereotyped into employment categories. Working-class men are employed in heavy, risky jobs, whilst middle-class men are employed in office or 'mental' work (Cornwall and Lindisfarne, 1994). The hazards of manual work, reflected in accidents at work and work-related diseases, are well known (Hart, 1985; Morgan et al., 1985). These hazards are reflected in the increased morbidity and mortality figures of men and may contribute to women's increased life expectancy over men's.

Men may also seek 'danger money' associated with hazardous jobs, work overtime, take a second part-time job or work in the informal economy, where there may be poor health and safety conditions.

Hart (1985) suggests that a stressor such as redundancy reduces the functioning of the immune system, making the person more susceptible to illness. The difference in men's ability to cope with stress may result from a lack of material resources and psychological support which assist coping behaviour.

Unemployment may affect men in one of two ways. For some, it can result in a feeling of worthlessness and a sense of failure, increasing stress and poverty. For others, it may lead to a reduction of stress caused by poor working conditions, offer financial gain through redundancy payments and allow more time for leisure activities.

Low income and low self-esteem resulting from unemployment may produce high morbidity and mortality because of mental or physical illness, shortened lifespan and a high rate of accidents (Fareed, 1994).

The effect of a prolonged period of unemployment on a man's self-image, impulsive behaviour and sexual relationship with his wife was noted by Tolson (1987). Long-term unemployment is a health hazard that must be recognized; mental health service input should be accessed where appropriate.

Low income, whether from unemployment or low-paid employment, also has an indirect effect on health and diet. The high sugar and low fibre content of the diets of social groups IV and V, compared with groups I and II, have been identifed as contributing to the higher rate of CHD amongst the manual classes (Townsend et al., 1992). Some of the variations may, however, be cultural rather than merely due to income.

Health care services

The male sex role stereotype demanding men to be healthy, strong and self-sufficient results in many men delaying seeking medical aid until they are acutely ill. Although it is recognized that men have high-risk health needs, there has been an absence of men demanding health care services despite high morbidity and mortality rates.

Local publicity resulted in only six men attending a London workshop for men (Matz, 1993). Matz concluded that, to meet the needs of men, an environment must be provided in which men feel safe enough to share their needs and feelings, and challenge oppressive aspects of sexism and homophobia.

The lower uptake of preventive health services amongst the manual classes has been explained in terms of their general orientation to the present and unwillingness to consider long-term benefits (Morgan et al., 1985), and is due more to cultural norms and voluntary behaviour choices than to material barriers such as limited access to the health services (Townsend et al., 1992; Fareed, 1994).

Health checks attract the 'worried well' and comfort the middle classes, who can afford to follow a reasonably healthy lifestyle. Those who would benefit most from health checks and health promotion receive it least; this is described as the inverse health care law. However, a health project in Glasgow has proved that working-class men can, and do, benefit from health care input once they overcome the traditional 'hard man' stereotype (McMillan, 1995).

Factors affecting men's decisions not to seek health care include the inconvenience of taking time off work for appointments and the potential loss of income from absenteeism, although work-related stress and competition to achieve career advancement may place men at particular risk of illness.

The quality of health care provision varies between the social classes. Whereas middle-class patients usually have high expectations of health outcome and are able to articulate their concerns, members of the lower social groups have shorter consultations and receive less information about their condition, referrals to specialist care being highest amongst patients in social class I and lowest in social class V (Morgan et al., 1985).

Health promotion is received more readily by the middle classes than manual workers, although the latter are said to be in greater need of lifestyle changes. Hart (1985) attributes this to middle-class socialization, which enables this group to adapt to changes in modern culture. Individuals from lower social classes find it more difficult to modify advice to fit their own perceived needs since most advice is generally based on the values and beliefs of the middle and upper classes (Tettersell and Luft, 1994).

> **Activity 5.1: Undertake, or refer to, a community or practice profile to identify priority issues for the health care of men in your practice.**

Well men

'Wellness' is peculiar to the individual and is difficult to define. One person may be in permanent pain but feel well because he can walk to the shops, whilst another will feel ill because of a headache.

Health prevention may be primary, secondary or tertiary. Primary prevention seeks to prevent the onset of disease through risk reduction, for example preventing hypertension by reducing alcohol consumption. Secondary prevention relates to the prevention of progression of a disease process, such as prescribing aspirin therapy following a heart attack or stroke. Tertiary health prevention involves measures to maximize health and minimize disability from a disease that cannot be cured. This may include lifestyle advice to stabilize blood sugar levels in diabetic patients.

It is important to determine the level of service the practice wishes to offer: a proactive approach to prevent disease, or a reactive approach to treat the condition. The latter offers easily accessible, quantifiable data, whereas the results of the former will not be apparent for many years (or decades).

Primary health care nurses are in an ideal position to offer a holistic approach to health. The health needs of men will differ according to their past and current lifestyles, whilst the time required to identify problems or promote health will vary. A well-man health check is an opportunity to offer structured health advice and can be incorporated into almost any consultation.

The benefits of cardiovascular screening and its subsequent interventions are controversial and often negative (Waller et al., 1990; Family Heart Study Group, 1994; Lindholm et al., 1995). However, structured health counselling has been shown to be a postive move towards the adoption of healthy lifestyle changes by men (Edgar, 1992).

Edwards (1996a) described the rationale behind a well-man programme that offers a holistic approach to men's health needs.

Although this is based on the Health of the Nation strategy (DoH, 1992), there are other important issues to be considered.

The term used to describe a well-man check is irrelevant, but the rationale behind each question or activity must be understood by the nurse and the patient for the intervention to be effective, informed and not merely a data collection activity.

General health

General health issues may include bladder and bowel changes or skin conditions. The well-man check allows men the opportunity to discuss any health concern, however apparently insignificant, and is an ideal opportunity to review any chronic disease, such as asthma or diabetes, which may save a future appointment.

Family history is non-modifiable, but many risk factors for premature morbidity and mortality can be modified. A healthy lifestyle usually includes non-smoking, moderate drinking, regular exercise and a healthy, balanced diet that maintains a body mass index of 20–25.

The DoH (1995) recognizes the benefits of regular exercise and advocates 30 minutes of moderate exercise, such as gardening, walking or manual work, a day. Fifty-eight per cent of men in a national survey cited lack of time as their main barrier to exercise (Office for National Statistics, 1995). This can be redressed by encouraging men in sedentary occupations to go for a walk at lunchtime, walk to the paper shop or take a brisk walk after tea. Manual workers often take sufficient unstructured exercise within their work to meet the recommendations.

The effectiveness of smoking cessation advice has been questioned by the OXCHECK study (Imperial Cancer Relief Fund, 1994a) but should still be an integral part of any health promotion programme.

The Office for National Statistics (ONS) reported that the majority of men find health professional advice about alcohol intake helpful, but that few men are offered advice (Office for National Statistics, 1995). The fear of losing a driving licence and/or employment following a drink-driving incident can be a major incentive to modify alcohol intake. Men with an acknowledged drink problem may wish to be referred for specialist advice.

It is unrealistic to advise on all the above issues in one short consultation. Further support should be offered for any area of concern, for example diet, weight, blood pressure or lipid levels.

Any screening process, including well-men checks, can be regarded in both positive and negative terms. Screening may confirm that an individual is in good health now, but it does not guarantee continued health. It could be argued that diagnosing a disease before it manifests with symptoms is beneficial to the patient. Conversely, it may increase stress and anxiety. Men who prefer not to be screened must have their views respected (see Chapter 1).

Key issues to be included in a holistic consultation can be seen in Box 5.1. This is intended to be not a comprehensive list but a reminder of the many facets of health that must be assessed.

Box 5.1: Factors to consider when assessing health

Factor	Risk
Family history	CHD, diabetes, familial hyperlipidaemia
Occupation	unemployment; stress from fear of redundancy or high-powered job; skin cancer from working outside; travel health, including STD's (see below); chemicals; hepatitis A or B (DoH, 1996b); other risks, including triggers for asthma, latex allergy and dermatitis; hearing loss
Use of recreational drugs	addiction
Hypertension	CHD, stroke
Diet	affects all aspects of health
Body mass index >30	diabetes, hypertension
Unplanned weight loss	medical referral needed
Exercise	lack of exercise can lead to obesity and CHD
Smoking	many cancers, respiratory disease
Alcohol abuse	cirrhosis of the liver, accidents at work and on the road, hypertension (DoH, 1992)
Glycosuria	diabetes
Proteinuria	renal disease, urinary infection
Haematuria	prostate disease, urinary infection, bladder disease
Travel (for leisure or work)	STD's, food hygiene, malaria, infectious diseases, accidents, skin cancer
Current chronic disease	compliance

Improving men's health

There is no doubt that health care workers must increase their efforts to target men's health in an attempt to reduce the health inequalities between both the sexes and the social classes, and to reduce morbidity and premature mortality caused by preventable diseases.

A flexible health care system that recognizes the constraints of some male occupations and permits men to talk openly about health issues will be a step towards empowering men to take more control of their health.

All men should be treated equally and offered sufficient information about diagnosis and proposed treatment on which to make an informed, autonomous decision about their care. Health promotion and health education should be similarly available. All health care should be independent of ethnicity, disability and social class.

A newspaper report stated that stress appears to be more common in the middle classes than manual workers (King, 1996), although men from all social groups present with stress-related illness in general practice. There may be a connection between stress and the present economic climate, which has resulted in men from all occupations living under a cloud of prospective unemployment.

Employment insecurity and an increase in marital breakdown, which often leads to a subsequent reduced income when a man has to support two households, is taking its toll on men across the social strata.

Health professionals play a major role in encouraging men to ignore the 'macho' image and allowing them to talk about, and share, their worries.

Summary

Ashton (1995) found that health promotion services providing male health clinics are neither acceptable nor convenient for men. Although men have historically been complacent or neglectful of their health, men's health appears to be receiving a higher profile in 1999 through media reports and journals such as 'Men's Health'. Health professionals must be abreast of current developments and discussions surrounding men's health if they wish to support men in the battle to increase their knowledge and awareness of men's health issues.

Seventy-three per cent of men questioned in a recent Gallup survey said that they would like to see men's health clinics becoming available (Men's Health Matters/Gallup, 1997). This is supported by the men in the author's practice, who are offered flexible, timed appointments for a well-man check, defaulters being in the minority. Anecdotal evidence indicates that men do appreciate someone being interested in their health; this is often stated during health checks. This applies to men of all ages where the practice does not operate an ageist policy. Although medical emphasis is placed on secondary prevention (e.g. post-cardiac event), it would appear logical to target men to prevent such events.

Health education enables an individual to exercise an informed choice when selecting the lifestyle he wishes to adopt. Nurses have a vital role in reducing the inequalities of health between men and women. Women who attend general practice for cervical smears will often receive a 'well-woman' health check. Men should be offered a similar regular, proactive health care service. This will identify some of the urinary problems faced by older men (see section on prostate cancer, below).

The risk factors for preventable disease should be explained and support for lifestyle modification offered. The individual will then have the knowledge with which to make an autonomous decision about his future lifestyle. Some men will inevitably continue to follow an unhealthy lifestyle; this is their choice and must be respected.

'Men's Health Review' (Lloyd, 1996) recommends further work and research to determine the range of factors that influence men's beliefs and behaviours. Health promotion can then be focused more accurately and effectively towards men.

Assumptions should never be made about men and their attitudes to health. Primary health prevention through well-men checks can reduce the morbidity and mortality of preventable diseases.

Activity 5.2: Carry out a small audit to assess the benefits of well-man checks in your practice.

Key points:

1. Men are socialized into a 'macho' image and are reluctant to express their emotional and personal needs.
2. Men do respond to structured health care counselling.
3. Primary health prevention is the first step towards reducing morbidity and premature mortality from preventable disease.

Sexual health of gay men

The health needs of gay men do not differ much from those of heterosexual men, although there are certain issues affecting gay men that must be understood if their health needs are to be met in a way conducive to effective health care and health promotion. Key issues will be discussed here. The reader who wishes to expand this knowledge is encouraged to contact gay support groups, attend sexual health clinics in his or her local area and read more widely about men's health.

Defining the patient group

The choice of terminology used to identify the patient group can be varied. It would be correct to use the term 'homosexual' instead of 'gay'. Bisexual men should also be included in the group. As men can and do identify with any of these terms, the most accurate definition of this patient group would be 'men who have sex with men'.

Some men who engage in sex with other men continue to regard themselves as heterosexual. These are usually married men who are constantly striving to suppress their homosexual feelings but still engage in homosexual acts in order to satisfy their sexual needs; they end up living what is effectively a double life that can often be full of guilt and stress-related health problems.

It is clear that it may not be as easy to identify gay men (men who have sex with men) as one might have thought.

The population

The gay population, just like any other, comes in all shapes and sizes from all backgrounds and social classes. Many people wrongly believe that all gay men live in London and other major cities. A sizeable percentage of gay men choose to move to the larger cities, where there is often less prejudice and a better gay scene, with cafés, pubs and night clubs which provide better opportunities to meet gay men. Other men may choose, or have no option but, to live in smaller cities, towns or villages that have no gay scene at all. It will not be easy to identify this client group, which often fails to comply with the stereotypical image that most people have of a gay man.

It must be acknowledged that many gay men will face prejudice, violence and rejection from others if they declare their sexuality, so it should not appear strange that they find it difficult to share this information with strangers, as well as friends and family.

Although there is very limited substantial research into the number of gay men in the UK, it is generally believed that one in every ten men has sex with men at some stage in his life. This includes any kind of sexual activity between two men (Box 5.2).

Although the Sexual Offences Act of 1967 legalized homosexual acts between two consenting adult males, there still remains much stigma against gay men despite gay role models such as sportsmen, musicians and MPs. Stigma and publicity are often attached to the

---

Box 5.2: Categories of sexual activity between two men

- Men who regularly have sex with different men
- Men who are in long-term monogamous relationships with other men
- Married men, who may also be parents, who may have occasional or regular sex with men
- Men who have had isolated sexual experiences with other men e.g. at school or university

---

'outing' (exposing a person against his will as being gay, often via the tabloid press) of gay or bisexual men.

Lifestyles

A brief look at the differing lifestyles of gay men will put their health needs into perspective. It has already been noted that 10 per cent of men will have some sexual activity with men during their lives and that homosexuality encompasses a wide cross-section of society.

Poverty

There is a myth that all gay men have high disposable incomes, good housing and employment. This is far from the truth. Within the gay community, there are many men and boys who live in very difficult circumstances, particularly men who have been rejected by their family and friends because of their sexuality. Rejection can lead to eviction from the family home with no further family contact. The adverse effects of poverty on health are well documented.

Male prostitution

Some young boys who have been rejected by their families end up working as 'rent boys' – male prostitutes who sell sex to men. Rent boys are as vulnerable to exploitation, sexually transmitted disease and rape as female prostitutes. Most people are not aware of the existence of rent boys, but wherever there are female prostitutes, there will often also be male prostitutes. Because of the prejudice they experience, male prostitutes are far less likely than female prostitutes to report abuse, assault and rape, and less likely to seek medical help.

Other health risks

The excessive use of recreational drugs, alcohol and cigarettes is commonplace within the club culture of gay life for some men. Many gay men train and tone their bodies in the quest for the perfect body that resembles the bronzed gods constantly seen in media advertising, which are believed to attract and satisfy partners. Whilst this activity can be of value to good health, there is often an abuse of steroids and an excessive use of sun beds, which brings associated health risks.

Older gay men often find themselves isolated. Some groups within the gay community are very insular and reject men who do not fit into their 'set'.

Bereavement

Commercial gay social life is primarily targeted towards the younger gay man who may have a high disposable income. Older men who have lost a partner through death can experience difficulty finding support in the community. They may also have lost family support because of previous rejection. Gay men need the same bereavement counselling and support services as heterosexual men and women but may find these difficult to access.

Vulnerability

Not all gay men, particularly married men who have sex with men, are able to, or choose to, go to gay pubs and clubs to meet people. They may choose to look for sex partners in places that can leave them vulnerable and in danger, such as 'cottages' (public toilets), cruising areas (parks, car parks and supermarkets), gyms and saunas.

Having so far painted a bleak picture of gay life, it must be remembered that many gay men live very ordinary, happy and healthy lives with the support of caring family and friends.

Adolescence

Homosexuality is often ignored in schools during sex education lessons because of Clause 28 of the Education Act (1987), which prevents schools promoting homosexual behaviour. This is unfortunately interpreted in many different ways, resulting in some young gay men being left in ignorance about where and how to get help in coming to terms with their sexuality, and how to live their lives in a healthy and safe way.

Within a climate of political correctness, this issue must be addressed in order to incorporate all areas of sexuality into health education programmes.

Coming out

'Coming out' is being open about one's sexuality. This takes on different meanings for different people. One person may be 'out' to family and friends, whilst another person may be 'out' to everyone. Some may be 'out' at work but not at home. It is therefore important to clarify what the person using the term understands it to mean and in what context he is using it.

From personal experience, coming out to my parents was the most difficult, frightening, challenging and also exciting and stimulating experience that I have ever had. It had to be done to liberate the self and be free to grow, but at the same time there is awareness of the danger of disclosure. There is an immense fear of rejection and the loss of all that is important to oneself and one's family. It is very difficult for a man to know where to go for help in coming to terms with his sexuality. Young and older men alike can be unsure of where to go for help.

Gay men regularly discuss their experiences, and differences, of coming out. I am always surprised by the number of men I meet who have not been able to 'come out' to their family and therefore end up living a life distant from their family. Unfortunately, some men who are able to pluck up the courage to 'come out' also end up living a life distant from their families following rejection.

There are limited postive images of gay men, especially for those who live in small towns. It may seem to the world that everywhere you look there are images of gay life – adverts on television for gay chat lines, gay men and gay lifestyles being portrayed in weekly soap programmes, and gay MPs living openly gay lives. However, life is still very different and so far removed from reality when a man has to tell his parents, siblings, aunts and uncles that he is not what they were expecting him to be. He is unable to fulfil the hopes and dreams they had for him to produce grandchildren and carry on the family name for generations to come. It is understandably difficult for parents to realize and accept that their son is gay, although the most important issue for parents is surely that their child is happy in life, whatever their destiny.

The parents of gay children may find it difficult to locate a sensitive person with whom they can discuss the problem of coming to terms with their son's sexuality. There are support groups in some of the larger cities, although these are not widespread.

It is still common for men who feel that they might be gay, but are unable to come to terms with their sexuality, to get married and have families before they are able finally to accept their own sexuality and find the strength to come out to themselves and possibly, at some stage, to their partners.

HIV, AIDS and hepatitis

HIV and AIDS were launched into the public arena in a blaze of media attention in early 1981. The response by the gay community to what is considered by many to have been the most successful public health campaign ever undertaken by the government was to have an immediate and dramatic effect on the way gay men lived their lives. Overnight, gay men's sexual habits changed. There was an instant increase in the use of condoms and the practice of safe and safer sex. This course of action has no doubt saved many lives and considerable finance.

Gay men are now victims of their own success. The initial dramatic increase in the number of people diagnosed with HIV were not as high as had been predicted by the government. This was due, in the main, to two factors in relation to the gay community: people chose not to be tested for fear of prejudice, and there was an initial decrease in the level of unsafe sex.

Unfortunately, there is now an increase in the number of HIV-positive younger gay males who, when questioned, say that they see HIV and AIDS as a disease that affects older gay men – those in their mid-thirties and over. Health professionals, in their role as health educators, must continue to provide appropriate information about HIV and AIDS.

It is estimated that, by the beginning of the next millenium, there will be between 30 and 40 million people infected with HIV throughout the world (WHO, 1993).

Although it is less publicized, men who have sex with men have an increased risk of contracting hepatitis through body fluids. They should therefore be offered vaccination as well as advice on safe sex. There are many books in print, and more appearing every week, on the topic of HIV/AIDS. Chapter 3 outlines infection control with respect to blood-borne viruses.

Male rape

Very few people are prepared or able to acknowledge that male rape takes place. Male rape is interpreted as a man being forced to have sex with a woman and is treated as something of a joke, something to be desired by 'real men'. Nothing could be further from the truth. Male rape, in this context, relates to men who are raped by other men. This may be anal penetration, violation or the abuse of an individual in a sexual manner.

Without doubt, a male rape victim will suffer considerable physical and emotional trauma. Few cases are reported to the police because the victim feels ashamed and may sometimes wrongly believe that he has been responsible for the attack. There has been limited confidence in the police handling of reported cases on the part of the gay community. During 1997, however, some police forces were working with gay communities to address this issue. This has resulted in an increase in the number of reported cases.

Men experience emotions similar to those of women following rape. Gay men may be reluctant to report the incident to the police for several reasons. They may have been cruising when attacked or they may not be 'out'; reported cases invariably make it into the tabloid press.

Male rape is not unique to gay men: straight men can also be attacked. The perpetrator of the crime does not necessarily go out to look for a gay man. His desires are usually similar to those of men who rape women, one of which is a need to control and have what they perceive to be power.

Men who have been in prison may have been subjected to rape and/or gang rape, in which more than one person is involved in the abuse. This can also occur in the sex rituals that some men experience as part of brutal initiation ceremonies into the military services.

A male rape victim may have nowhere to turn for help. The specialist counselling services and telephone helplines that are so valuable to the female victim do not exist for male victims. The understanding and support available from some police forces is limited because of ignorance and prejudice.

Confidentiality

An assessment of the sexual health needs of gay and bisexual men, and men who have sex with men, living in the Northallerton area was researched and compiled by Yorkshire MESMAC Sexual Health Project (Doyle and Gale, 1996). One of the main reasons why men did not attend health centres and surgeries for their health needs was that they had no confidence that confidentiality would be maintained in relation to their sexuality. Confidentiality is integral to all aspects of health care and must not be breached (see Chapter 1).

An excellent example of a forward-thinking surgery is the DOCS surgery in the heart of Manchester's gay quarter, which recognized that 25 per cent of its clients were gay. The surgery has adjusted to meet the needs of both gay and straight patients by creating an environment that is acceptable to all the clients. Posters, leaflets and comprehensive information displays address health issues for clients. Information on post-rape counselling and support includes both male and female rape.

Gay patients who are in a relationship can register as a family and are recognized as such. The team have clearly been able to gain the confidence of their patients, who feel that the surgery is a safe environment, one in which confidentiality will not be breached.

The role of the practice nurse

As previously mentioned, the health needs of gay men do not differ greatly from those of heterosexual men, except in the key areas discussed briefly above. Gay men are often more receptive to health promotion than straight men. Good health, including fitness in order to achieve an attractive body, as discussed above, tends to have a high profile within the gay community.

The practice nurse is ideally placed to play a key role in meeting the health needs of gay men (Box 5.3). The aim is not to be able to identify or encourage a gay client to disclose his sexuality, but to create an environment in which the man will be comfortable to attend for help and support for all aspects of physical and/or mental health related to his sexuality.

Box 5.3: Role of the practice nurse

- To create a non-judgemental surgery environment
- To develop an action plan for the primary health care team
- As a health educator on all aspects of a healthy lifestyle
- As a resource for information about support groups
- To liaise with the health promotion department
- To liaise with local groups
- To develop a resource folder of contacts and addresses
- To refer to mental health services where appropriate

Primary health care team commitment

The first major task to overcome is that of obtaining agreement from the other team members to be involved in developing an action plan to meet the needs of this client group. Within the team, there will be many different levels of understanding and prejudice with regard to men who have sex with men; these must be acknowledged. Team commitment is essential for any action plan to work.

If there are 2000 adult males in a practice population, 200 will at some time or other have sex with another man. This emphasizes that these health care issues cannot be ignored.

The action plan can involve a simple approach that involves little time and effort:

- Review poster displays.
- Review the available leaflets.

Health promotion

The role of the practice nurse as a health promoter is ideally suited to providing the appropriate information about HIV and AIDS, which was mentioned above. The information should be appropriate to all clients, regardless of sexual orientation, but if a leaflet does not appear to be specific to gay men, it will be left on the shelf.

A visit to the health promotion department will reveal a collection of posters and leaflets on all the topics that have been briefly discussed in this section. Information relating to adolescence and sex education – for example, on being gay, coming out and safe and safer sex – should be included.

Posters and leaflets need to be displayed with other health promotion literature so patients can pick them up unobtrusively. The knowledge that someone can see what is selected may deter some people from choosing leaflets. It is possible to measure the demand for certain pieces of literature by displaying a numbered amount.

Posters should depict positive images of gay life rather than refer to HIV and AIDS. Additional posters and leaflets in the nurses' and doctors' rooms may be more accessible to some patients.

Local groups

For more comprehensive information and a greater insight, local HIV and AIDS groups and support groups for gay men and the parents of gay children can be contacted; their addresses should be found in the telephone directory. Some of these groups will be willing to come to the surgery or let nurses visit them to develop a knowledge base. Posters and leaflets will also be available from these groups.

Training

It will be necessary to assess training needs for staff once the proposed input has been discussed and the specific needs identified. It may be appropriate to develop counselling skills for post-male rape victims, those suffering bereavement and the parents of gay males. If these services are provided by other agencies, a support and referral network can be developed.

Summary

The health needs of gay men include all the social and physical issues that were discussed in the first section of this chapter.

Whilst some gay men will be very comfortable with their sexuality and assertive about their health needs, they may not be able or ready to declare their sexuality to a stranger in the middle of the surgery. It may therefore be difficult to identify and assess the health needs of this population (see Chapter 4).

It is important to create an environment in which men who have sex with men, regardless of whether they are 'out' gay men or men who have not yet been able fully to come to terms with their sexuality, will be able to recognize that the nurse's place of work is one in which they will be welcome, well cared for and respected. It will be a place where they can get help and advice or be directed to other agencies, and it will offer the same level of service that is offered to other members of society.

Key points:

1. One in ten men experiences sex with another man.
2. Gay men often fail to comply with their stereotypical image.
3. Gay men usually respond positively to health education.
4. It is often necessary to seek appropriate and effective information and support for gay men from sources outside the NHS.

Testicular and prostate cancer

Testicular cancer is the most common form of cancer in young men, occurring mostly in those aged between 15 and 49 (Imperial Cancer Reseach Fund, 1997), whilst four times as many men die from prostate cancer than women from cervical cancer in England and Wales (Willis, 1993).

Ashton (1995) reported that the NHS does not regard men's health as a key issue. This is supported by the Health of the Nation targets (DoH, 1992), which made no mention of reducing testicular or prostate cancer. Men must be involved in their own health screening and, through health promotion, be made aware that they are not immune to testicular and prostate disease. This section aims to provide the reader with an insight into the complexity of issues surrounding the aetiology and screening of these diseases.

Testicular cancer

Prevalence

Testicular cancer is still uncommon, with just over 1500 new cases and about 90 deaths per year in the UK (Imperial Cancer Research Fund, 1997). The risk of dying from testicular cancer has decreased over the past 20 years, 130 deaths a year being cited by the Cancer Research Campaign (1991) as the previous figure, although the risk of developing this disease has nearly doubled and is still increasing.

Aetiology

Although the aetiology of testicular cancer is uncertain, socio-economic status and factors of modern life are thought to be contributory (Cancer Research Campaign, 1991). Genetic, hormonal and environmental factors are also thought to contribute to the development of testicular cancer, although supporting evidence is said to be lacking (Summers, 1995). The epidemiology unit in Oxford has investigated hormone levels in mothers whose pregnancy resulted in a child with undescended testicles, in an effort to learn more about the genetic mechanisms involved in the development of these tumours and possible ways of reducing risks (Imperial Cancer Research Fund, 1994b).

Cancer Research Campaign (1991) research highlighted geographical variations in the incidence of disease. Testicular cancer is more common in Northern Europe and generally rare in non-Caucasian men. Statistics highlight a consistent reduction in black, compared with white, American men, suggesting a genetic component to the disease. However, the rates rise in African and other non-Caucasian migrants to the USA, suggesting the influence of some environmental factor(s) (Rosella, 1994).

As early as 1921, British mortality rates of testicular cancer were known to be highest amongst professional, administrative and clerical workers, and lowest among manual workers (Pike and Chilvers, 1992). The young age of onset of this cancer, and the social mobility of many men during their working lives, has persistently cast doubt on the role of occupation in aetiology.

Although there are no known causes for the rising incidence of testicular cancer, possible factors have been proposed (Box 5.4).

Box 5.4: Suggested risk factors for testicular cancer (Cancer Research Campaign, 1991; Imperial Cancer Research Fund, 1997)

- Past medical history of:
  - undescended testicles increases the risk five-fold; if corrected before the age of 10 years, this is no longer a risk factor
  - inguinal hernia
  - testicular torsion
  - testicular trauma
  - mumps/orchitis
  - prenatal exposure to oestrogen
- Other factors:
  - age 15–49 years
  - white
  - early age of puberty
  - rare familial syndromes
  - close family relatives (brother or father) with testicular cancer increases the risk ten-fold
  - wearing tight underwear
  - central heating
  - hot baths

Symptoms

Testicular cancer usually presents as a painless enlargement of one testicle (Box 5.5). The initial absence of pain, combined with a lack of knowledge, often causes men to delay seeking medical advice. Very rarely, the tumour may disappear and the first symptom is backache from metastases.

Diagnosis

Only a small minority of men require referral and treatment. The doctor will examine and reassure a man who has a benign lump; intrascrotal masses in young men can be secondary to non-malignant disease. An ultrasound will suggest a cancerous growth, which is confirmed after biopsy and microscopic examination. In some cases, diagnosis can be made only by surgical exploration.

Box 5.5: Symptoms of testicular cancer

In the early stages of the disease, the man might notice:
- a painless enlargement of the testicle;
- a vague 'heaviness' in the scrotum.

As the disease spreads, he may feel:
- a dull ache in the groin or lower abdomen;
- backache;
- an alteration in the firmness of the testes;
- a hard, small irregular lump on palpation when the cancer has infiltrated to the lymph nodes or bones.

Testicular cancers may be germ cell tumours, seminomas (usually malignant), teratomas (benign) or of mixed aetiology. Teratomas usually affect men aged 15–30 years; seminomas are more common in men aged 30–50 years.

Treatment

Testicular cancer is highly susceptible to modern treatments, and the vast majority of men are cured, with an overall survival rate of over 90 per cent (Imperial Cancer Research Fund, 1997). However, if treatment is delayed, the disease can be fatal (Schaufele, 1988). For men who are identified and treated early on, even when the cancer has progressed to a metastatic (advanced) stage, cure rates of 60 per cent have been achieved (Cancer Reseach Campaign, 1991).

Surgery will normally be carried out to remove the affected testicle (orchidectomy); cancer of both testicles is rare. Chemotherapy is usually given for metastatic spread, whilst radiotherapy may be used for a few men in the early stages of disease. Occasionally, surgery is required to remove any residual lumps following treatment.

The reader is referred to Peate (1997) for details of survival rates for differing cancers.

Fertility

The loss of one testicle *per se* does not affect fertility, although treatment with radiotherapy or chemotherapy can affect fertility for 12–24 months (Imperial Cancer Research Fund, 1997). There is no evidence of any genetic risk from treatment in children fathered by men treated for testicular cancer.

Altered body image

A man who loses a testicle, for whatever reason, can suffer shame and distress, with a psychological loss of self-esteem (Blackmore,

1989). He may feel less masculine, less virile and less able to perform sexually, although the latter may be perceived loss of sexual function. The anxiety and depression that follow orchidectomy can last for several years.

Testicular self-awareness

Testicular cancer is still relatively uncommon compared with other cancers, but there is clearly a need for a change in attitude to the role of men in society.

Male body awareness is, in general, very low, and few men are taught to recognize the warning signs of testicular disease, which results in a delay in seeking medical advice (Bell, 1990, Bassett, 1993). Forrester (1986) suggested that the idea of testicular self-examination (TSE) is, to many men, somehow unmanly or linked to homosexuality or masturbation.

Men need a clearer understanding of the role of TSE and its importance in reducing morbidity and mortality through the early detection of cancer. There is no normal testicular size or shape; all men, from the onset of puberty, should be aware of what is normal for them. This parallels the advice given to women for breast awareness.

TSE (Figures 5.1–5.3) should be carried out routinely. It is most easily done after a warm bath or shower when the scrotal sac is relaxed. The testes should feel firm and smooth. Any change or irregularity should be discussed with a doctor. The majority of lumps found on TSE are benign, and men must be reassured that it is uncommon for a lump to be malignant.

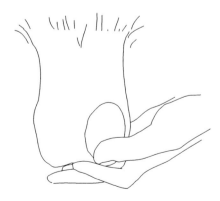

Figure 5.1: Roll the testis between the thumb and forefingers. Check along the length of the epididymis for any swellings.

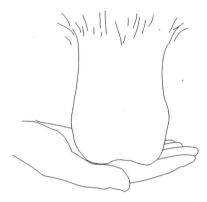

Figure 5.2: Check the weight of the testes with the palm of the hand.

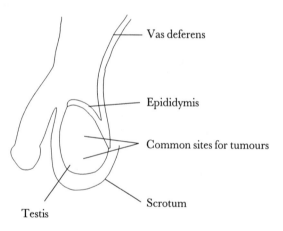

Figure 5.3: Diagram of the position of the testes.

Men need to be reassured that it is normal to be interested in one's health and that self-awareness is vital to detect any disease at an early stage. This is relevant to all aspects of men's health, including skin changes, bowel changes or urinary symptoms.

Role of the practice nurse

Evidence suggests that the early detection of testicular cancer improves morbidity and mortality. TSE is a simple, effective screening procedure that is easily taught and practised. Tugwell (1996) demonstrated the benefits of teaching TSE in her audit of military personnel, although a minority of men thought that this topic should not be discussed.

TSE is as controversial as breast self-examination. Morris (1996) argues that TSE unduly creates anxiety, inevitable false positives and an increased number of general practitioner consultations and hospital referrals. These are pertinent issues for any screening process, but they have not prevented women's health screening progressing and should not prevent the promotion of men's health.

Nurses must feel comfortable, and not embarrassed, in discussing this procedure with young men. It is inevitable that some young men will be embarrassed by any mention of their genitalia, but a professional approach by the nurse can defuse this embarrassment.

Literature reinforcing the information can be read at leisure and shared with friends and family. TSE leaflets should be readily available for men and women (wives, mothers, girlfriends, partners) in the surgery. It has been suggested that men can identify with photographic visual aids, which are more realistic than diagrammatic aids, although the sensitivity of cultural issues must not be ignored (Peate, 1997).

The practice nurse who does not feel confident reassuring a man about and discussing with him his future sexual function and fertility should refer to a community psychiatric nurse, specialist nurse or psychosexual counsellor (Blackmore, 1989).

Testicular awareness (Box 5.6) should be included in all health promotion/well-men health checks, particularly for men under 49 years of age. Young men must be alerted to the potential risks associated with wearing tight underwear and tight trousers, and having hot baths. Men should be allowed the opportunity to take some responsibility for their own health.

Box 5.6: Role of the nurse in testicular self-awareness

- Ask about past medical/family history – is there a risk factor?
- Determine level of awareness of testicular disease
- Discuss TSE if appropriate
- Reinforce with leaflets if required
- Emphasize that most lumps are benign
- Encourage the man to seek medical advice if there are any changes in the testes
- Advise on a healthy lifestyle

Summary

In order to reduce morbidity and mortality rates in young men, education in TSE should begin at an early age, particularly if there are known risk factors (Rosella, 1994). Men should be reassured that lumps are rarely malignant. A neurotic man who overpalpates his testes may develop 'self-palpation orchitis', which can mimic referred pain (Holland et al., 1994).

To improve the process and raise awareness, access to health education services within the primary care, secondary education and employment sectors must encourage males to be more conscious of, and take more responsibility for, their health.

Ganog and Markeritz (1987) reported that young men frequently go out of their way to avoid any sort of health education and actively neglect their own health. The authors' experiences of health education with young men does not support this view in the late 1990s, although the uptake of health services will, of course, vary between and within regions and general practices.

Community nurses are ideally placed to initiate health promotion services that play a major role in educating men to be more conscious about their health, and to raise the profile of testicular cancer. TSE/self-awareness is a cheap screening method that can reduce the morbidity and mortality caused by this common disease.

Prostate cancer

Prostate cancer has provoked an intense debate in recent years as a result of incomplete knowledge about the disease and its treatment (Scardino, 1994). Three main areas of concern and controversy surrounding prostate cancer are risk, screening and management (Lloyd, 1996, p. 12). Nurses will encounter many men with prostastic symptoms in general practice and will be expected to answer questions relating to the tests for, and management of, prostate cancer. When the arguments for and against prostate screening have been examined, the nurse may feel more competent to answer some of these questions.

Incidence

Cancer of the prostate is the third most common cause of cancer death amongst men in the UK, after lung cancer and large bowel cancer (University of York, 1997), resulting in over 9500 deaths in the UK in 1992 (Buck, 1995). However, many men have a slow-growing cancer that does not spread, resulting in men dying *with* the disease rather than *from* it (Willis, 1993).

Of the 10 per cent of men who have clinically detected prostate cancer, 3 per cent will die from the disease (Roberts, 1994). Although prostate cancer can and does occur in men in their 40s, approximately 85 per cent of prostate cancer patients are over 65 years of age (Buck, 1995). Prostate cancer is characteristically a disease of old men, although the incidence of, and mortality from, prostate cancer is said to be increasing faster than can be attributed solely to the ageing population (Schroder, 1995).

One in ten men will have the disease by the age of 85, with a 5-year survival rate of 28 per cent if the patient has distant metastases at diagnosis (Woolf, 1994).

Aetiology

There is no one specific factor causing prostate cancer. Suggested risk factors are summarized in Box 5.7.

Box 5.7: Risk factors for prostate cancer (Imperial Cancer Research Fund, 1994b; Dearnaley, 1994)

- Risk increases with age
- More common in black men than white
- Family history of breast or prostate cancer
- Exposure to cadmium or radiation
- Vasectomy
- Benign prostatic hypertrophy
- Weak evidence for an association with a high-fat, low-green vegetable diet, sexual activity, the number of sexual partners and a history of sexually transmitted diseases

---

Diagnosis

Presenting symptoms that relate to enlargement of the prostate gland usually involve bladder outflow obstruction, resulting in difficulty in passing urine, although in most cases the enlargement is benign. Men who have prostate cancer may also be asymptomatic. Men are advised to seek medical advice if they have difficulty passing urine, get up regularly in the night to pass urine or pass blood in their urine.

The disease is diagnosed by a urologist only after several investigations.

Prostate-specific antigen

Measurement of the level of prostate-specific antigen (PSA) is a blood test specific for prostate tissue rather than prostate cancer; the PSA can show false positive and false negative results for cancer. Although PSA measurement has been shown to pick up 60 per cent of well-developed cancers (Catalona et al., 1991), two-thirds of men who have higher levels of PSA do not have cancer (University of York, 1997).

Up to 1 per cent of men under the age of 50 with a normal PSA level will go on to develop invasive cancer in the next 10 years, with a slightly higher preponderance of older men (University of York, 1997).

Digital rectal examination

On rectal examination, a normal prostate gland feels smooth, rubbery and mobile. A prostate cancer may feel enlarged, hard and fixed. This is, however, not an accurate assessement when taken in isolation: apparent cancers have been found to be benign, and smooth glands have been malignant (personal communication).

Transrectal ultrasound and biopsy

Transrectal ultrasound (TRUS) is performed via a rectal probe. A needle biopsy may be taken during this procedure to assess the grade and and type of cancer. Complications of needle biopsy include infection and prolonged rectal bleeding.

TRUS is an expensive procedure, especially if used with needle biopsy, and is thought to be unable to detect 10–20 per cent of cancers located in the transitional zone (Narayan, 1992).

Treatment

There are several treatment options for localized prostatic cancer (Box 5.8).

The effectiveness of radical prostatectomy or pelvic irradiation has been questioned by Litwin and deKernion (1994). Radical prostatectomy and radiation can result in incontinence, bowel injury, stricture and impotence (Adami et al., 1994; Handley and Stuart, 1994; Pomfret, 1995). Figures for impotency vary. Dearnaley (1993) reported that, with skilled surgery, over 95 per cent of men retain continence, whilst 50 per cent will retain potency. However, these figures conflict with data from the University of York (1997) (Table 5.1).

Box 5.8: Treatment options for prostate cancer

- Watchful waiting – waiting to see how the disease progresses before choosing an invasive treatment option
- Radical prostatectomy
- Radiation

Hanbury and Sethia (1995) reported that 2.9 per cent of men in their study were totally impotent following transurethral prostatectomy, whilst 17.5 per cent had reduced potency. The risk of impotence was directly related to capsular perforation at the time of surgery. Surgery is generally restricted to younger, fit men who have no lymph gland involvement (Dearnaley, 1994).

Table 5.1: Outcome following surgery and radiation per 1000 men with prostate cancer (University of York, 1997)

Outcome	Treatment with surgery	Treatment with radiation
Die because of treatment	3–20	2–5
Experience impotence	200–850	400–670
Develop urinary incontinence	10–850	10–30

Watchful waiting is precisely what it says: monitoring of the PSA level and symptoms to assess the progress of the disease. Active treatment is undertaken if the PSA levels rise or symptoms worsen.

Most prostatic cancers regress when treated by the conventional first-line approach of androgen withdrawal, although the remission is temporary (Muir and Stratton, 1993). Cancers that shrink in response to male hormone deprivation will subsequently recur at a mean of 15–18 months later. The reader is referred to the 'British National Formulary' for details of the range of available therapies and their side-effects.

Screening

Screening identifies diseases in an asymptomatic person. Prostate screening has been defined as 'the testing of all men within the population who meet certain criteria as part of a community health programme' (Buck, 1995). Screening is controversial, mainly because of the financial cost to the NHS in comparison with the extended life expectancy and the increased anxiety for the patient.

Early prostate cancer is usually asymptomatic and may be detected by digital rectal examination or PSA testing. PSA estimation is said to improve the detection of prostate cancer confined to the gland by as much as 78 per cent compared with digital rectal examination (Schroder, 1995). The tandem use of digital rectal examination and PSA testing for primary screening has proved to be effective, although there is a need for a clear explanation of treatment options at the time of diagnosis of the cancer (Howe, 1994). TRUS results in many false positives and should therefore be viewed as being complemetary to digital rectal examination (Buck, 1995).

The University of York (1997) has stated that little good quality research has been carried out on prostate cancer screening and that the benefits of breast cancer screening do not apply to prostate cancer.

What do men want?

Handley and Stuart (1994) report that employing shared decision-making to determine whether PSA screening is to be used suggests that patients may choose not to be screened by PSA testing once they are fully informed of the risks and benefits of screening. This contradicts Howe (1994), who suggests that a majority of patients will choose surgery or radiation in the hope of achieving a cure despite the risks of significant side-effects.

It has been reported that many men want to know if they have a disease, even if there is no proven treatment (Woolf, 1994). Ninety-two per cent of men across all age groups in a 1997 Gallup survey, once they were aware that earlier detection would help to prevent future kidney problems, said that they would go for prostate screening if it were easily available (MHM/Gallup, 1997).

Role of the practice nurse

The role of the practice nurse will vary between practices. A practice that runs prostate clinics will optimize nurses' skills in this area. Prostate clinics may be used to identify men with bladder outflow obstruction and follow up men who are 'watchful waiting' cases, employing shared care with a urologist (Cutinha et al., 1996). A realistic role for the nurse includes:

* encouraging men to seek early advice for urinary symptoms such as nocturia, difficulty in starting to pass urine, a poor stream or haematuria;

- the identification of bladder outflow obstruction through sensitive questioning during routine consultations;
- referring to the general practitioner for reassurance or investigations and/or simply reassurance;
- explaining proposed investigations and interpreting the results if necessary;
- explaining proposed treatment options and outcomes if asked;
- acting as a source of information, leaflets, videos and support;
- giving hormone injections.

The nurse may be expected to undertake any or all of the above roles, depending on his or her individual competence.

Summary

The increasing number and variety of health-related articles that are published in the daily and weekend newspapers inevitably send men scuttling to the doctor or nurse for reassurance or information about different diseases, including prostate disease. The nurse must have unbiased information to present to a man who requests a test for prostate cancer. Edwards (1996b) argues that men should be given sufficient information to make an informed decision to be screened (see Chapter 1).

Discomfort from bladder flow obstruction may be caused by a benign tumour, so men must be reassured of this more common option. Prostate cancer investigations may well be initiated by the doctor when a man presents with urinary symptoms. A combination of a raised PSA level and abnormal digital rectal examination findings will probably result in referral to a urologist for further investigations and possible treatment. These men may appreciate information leaflets, videos and support while they await their appointment and during their 'watchful waiting' period.

By the year 2010, it is predicted that prostate cancer will be the most common cause of cancer death in men (Alexander and Boyle, 1995) as the life expectancy of men continues to rise. Screening for prostate cancer may then be considered beneficial.

Key points:

1. Screening for testicular and prostate cancer is controversial.
2. Testicular cancer, although uncommon, affects young men.
3. Most men will die with prostate cancer rather than from it.
4. Nurses must be informed in order to educate.

References

Adami H, Baron JA, Rothman KJ (1994) Ethics of a prostate cancer screening trial. Lancet 343: 958-9.

Alexander FE, Boyle P (1995) The rise in prostate cancer – myth or reality. In Kirby M, (1997) Primary Health Care Vol 7 No3: 17–20.

Armstrong D (1994) An Outline of Sociology as Applied to Medicine 4th ed. Oxford: Butterworth Heineman.

Ashton R (1995) Men are a low priority in the NHS. Which Way to Health August: 112.

Bassett C (1993) Pay attention to the testes. Practice Nurse 5(14): 956–7.

Bell I (1990) Testicular self-examination. Nursing Times 86(9): 38–40.

Blackmore C (1989) Altered images. Nursing Times 85(12): 36–9.

Blaxter M (1990) Health and Lifestyles. London: Tavistock/Routledge.

Bone MR, Bebbington AC, Jagger C, Morgan K, Nicholaas G (1995) Health Expectancy and its Uses. London: HMSO.

Buck AC (1995) Prostate Cancer. Questions and Answers. Hampshire: Merit Publishing.

Cancer Research Campaign (1991) Testicular Cancer Factsheet 16.1–16.4. London: CRC.

Catalona WJ et al. (1991) Measurement of prostate specific antigen in serum as a screening test for prostate cancer. Cited in Lloyd T (1996) Men's Health Review. Prepared on Behalf of the Men's Health Forum, p. 13. London: RCN.

Cornwall A, Lindisfarne N (1994) Dislocating Masculinity. Comparative Ethnographies. London: Routledge.

Cutinha PE, Potts KL, Rosario DJ, Hastie KJ, Moore KTH, Chapple CR (1996) Prospective audit of the use of a prostate clinic. British Journal of Urology 78: 733–6.

Dearnaley DP (1993) Clinical overview. Lancet 342: 904–5.

Dearnaley DP (1994) Cancer of the prostate. British Medical Journal 308: 780–4.

Department of Health (1992) The Health of the Nation: A Strategy for Health in England. London: HMSO.

Department of Health (1993) On the State of the Public Health 1992. London: HMSO.

Department of Health (1995) The Health of the Nation. More People More Active More Often: Physical Activity in England. A Consultative Paper. London: HMSO.

Department of Health (1996a) Health-related Behaviour: An Epidemiological Overview. London: HMSO.

Department of Health (1996b) Immunisation against Infectious Diseases. London: HMSO.

Doyle T, Gale D (1996) An Assessment of the Sexual Health Needs of Gay, Bisexual and Men who Have Sex with Men Living and Working in the Northallerton Area. Leeds: Yorkshire MESMEC.

Edgar M (1992) Collaboration between a district health authority and a family health services authority: structured health counselling within general practices. In Health Education Authority, Beating Heart Disease in the 1990's: A Strategy for 1990–1995. London: HEA. 125–31.

Edwards M (1996a) Setting up a well man programme. Nursing in General Practice 2(1): 4–5.

Edwards M (1996b) Prostate cancer: to screen or not? Practice Nursing 7(3): 40–2.

Family Heart Study Group (1994) Randomised controlled trial evaluating cardio-vascular screening and intervention in general practice: principal results of the British Family Heart Study. British Medical Journal 308: 313–20.

Fareed A (1994) Equal rights for men. Nursing Times 90(5): 26–9.

Forrester DA (1986) Myths of masculinity impact upon men's health. Nursing Clinics of North America 21: 15–23.

Ganog WH, Markeritz J (1987) Young men's knowledge of testicular cancer and behavioural intentions towards testicular self-examination. Patient Education and Counselling 9: 251–61.

Hanbury DC, Sethia KK (1995) Erectile function following transurethral prostate-ctomy. British Journal of Urology 75: 12–13.

Handley MR, Stuart ME (1994) The use of prostate specific antigen for prostate cancer: a managed case perspective. Journal of Urology 152: 1689–92.

Hart N (1985) The Sociology of Health and Medicine. Ormskirk: Causeway.

Health Education Authority (1990) Beating Heart Disease in the 1990's: A Strategy for 1990–1995. London: HEA.

Holland JM, Feldman JL, Gilbert HC (1994) Phantom orchalgia. Journal of Urology 152: 2291–3.

Howe RJ (1994) Prostate cancer: a patient's perspective. Journal of Urology 152: 1700–3.

Imperial Cancer Research Fund (1994a) Effectiveness of health checks conducted by nurses in primary care: results of the OXCHECK study after one year. British Medical Journal 308: 308–12.

Imperial Cancer Research Fund (1994b) Testicular Cancer Fact Sheet. London: ICRF.

Imperial Cancer Research Fund (1997) Testicular Cancer Fact Sheet. London: ICRF.

King A (1996) Living well but still lazy after all these years. Daily Telegraph 2 January: 4.

Lindholm LH, Ekbom T, Dash C, Eriksson M, Tibblin G, Schersten P (on behalf of the CELL Study Group) (1995) The impact of health care advice given in primary care on cardiovascular risks. British Medical Journal 310: 1105–9.

Litwin MS, deKernion JB (1994) Editorial: Perspectives on the problems of prostate cancer. Journal of Urology 152: 1680–1.

Lloyd T (1996) Men's Health Review. Prepared on Behalf of the Men's Health Forum. London: RCN.

McMillan I (1995) The life of Riley. Nursing Times 91(48): 27–8.

Matz R (1993) Men, Masculinity and Male Health. London: Albany Health Project.

Men's Health Matters/Gallup (1997) Men's Health Matters in the Nineties. Report of the Survey. London: MHM.

Morgan M, Calnan M, Manning N (1985) Sociological Approaches to Health and Medicine. London: Routledge.

Morris J (1996) The case against TSE. Nursing Times 92(33): 41.

Muir G, Stratton M (1993) Mechanism of hormone independence. Lancet 342: 903–4.

Narayan P (1992) Neoplasms of the prostate gland. Cited in Lloyd T (1996) Men's Health Review. Prepared on Behalf of the Men's Health Forum, p. 13. London: RCN.

Nicholson J (1993) Men and Women. How Different are They, New 2 Edn. Oxford: Oxford University Press.

Office for National Statistics (1995) Health in England 1995: What People Know, What People Think, What People Do. London: HMSO.

Peate I (1997) Testicular cancer: the importance of effective health education. British Journal of Nursing 6(6): 311–16.

Pike C, Chilvers MC (1992) Cancer risk in the undescending testicles, European Urology Update Service 1: 14-79.

Pomfret I (1995) Incontinence: the man's story. Practice Nursing 6(16): 37–9.

Roberts RG (1994) Prostate cancer, screening and the generalist physician. Journal of Urology 152: 1693–4.

Rosella JD (1994) Testicular cancer health. Education on integrative review. Journal of Advanced Nursing 20: 666–71.

Scardino PT (1994) Problem of prostate cancer. Journal of Urology 152: 1677–8.

Schaufele B (1988) Teaching testicular self-examination. Professional Nurse 9(10): 409–11.

Schroder FH (1995) Detection of prostate cancer. British Medical Journal 310: 140–1.

Summers E (1995) Vital signs. Nursing Times 91(25): 46–7.

Tettersell M, Luft S (1994) Lifestyle influences on client health. In Luft S, Smith M (Eds) Nursing in General Practice, London: Chapman & Hall: 37–57.

Tolson A (1987) The Limits of Masculinity. London: Routledge.

Townsend P, Davidson N, Whitehead M (1992) Inequalities in Health. London: Penguin.

Tugwell M (1996) Testicular self-examination. Primary Health Care 6(5): 18–19, 21.

University of York (1997) Screening for Prostate Cancer: The Evidence. Effectiveness Matters. York: NHS Centre for Reviews and Dissemination.

Waller D, Agass M, Mant D, Coulter A, Fuller A, Jones L (1990) Health checks in general practice: another example of inverse care. British Medical Journal 300: 1115–18.

Willis J (1993) Dying of embarrassment. Nursing Times 89(27): 22–3.

Woolf ST (1994) Public health perspective: the health policy implications of screening for prostate cancer. Journal of Urology 152: 1685–8.

World Health Organization (1993) Press release WHO/69, 7 September. Geneva: WHO.

Further reading

Naidoo J, Wills J (1994) Health Promotion: Foundations for Practice. London: Baillière Tindall.

Scrambler G (1991) Sociology as Applied to Medicine, 3rd Edn. London: Baillière Tindall.

Pratt R (1995) HIV and AIDS. A Strategy for Nursing Care, 4th Edn. London: Edward Arnold.

Useful addresses

British Medical Association Foundation for AIDS,
BMA House,
Tavistock Square,
London WC1H 9JP
Tel: 0171–383 6345   Helpline: 0171–383 6315

Offers information, advice and publications to medical professionals.

CRUISAID
Livingstone House,
11 Carteret Street,
London SW1H 9DJ
Tel: 0171–976 8200

Also in Dutch, French and Italian; Tel: +44 171 976 8100.

CRUISAID Scotland
25 Queensferry Street,
Edinburgh EH2 4QS
Tel: 0131–220 4033

National fundraising, grants and awareness.

Gay Men Fighting AIDS (GMFA)
Unit 42, Eurolink Centre,
49 Effra Road,
London SW2 1BZ
Tel: 0171–738 7140

Also in French; Tel:+44 171 738 6872

Gay men's work: prevention, outreach, support, information, research and advocacy.

HIV and AIDS Nursing National Forum
Royal College of Nursing,
20 Cavendish Square,
London W1M 0AB
Tel: 0171–647 3740

Special interest group for nurses that provides information and resources. Participates in the formulation of RCN policy and participates in national lobbying.

Imperial Cancer Research Fund
PO Box 123,
Lincoln's Inn Fields,
London WC2A 3PX
Tel: 0171–242 0200

Wallace House,
Maxwell Place,
Stirling FK8 1JU
Tel: (01786) 479137

London Lesbian and Gay Switchboard
PO Box 7324,
London N1 9QS
Tel: 0171–837 6768   Helpline 0171–837 7324

Lesbian and gay helpline: advice, information, referrals, counselling and publications.

London Lighthouse
111–117 Lancaster Road,
London W11 1QT
Tel: 0171–792 1200

Residential and support centre: drop-in, information, advice, counselling, support, documentation centre, complementary therapies, medical care, training, research, policy development, home support and newsletter.

Men's Health Matters
Blythe Hall,
100 Blythe Road,
London W14 0AB

Provides leaflets on prostate problems. Please send SAE.

Network of Sexwork Projects
c/o AHRTAG,
Farringdon Road,
London EC1M 3JB
Tel: 0171–609 0112

Sex workers' organization: information and advice.

Chapter 6
Women's health

Georgina Paget, Gudrun Limbrick and
Jean Crutchley

Women's health appears to have dominated much of the health-related data in nursing texts. This chapter examines three areas of women's health that have received less coverage and of which the practice nurse may have insufficient knowledge to address the topic confidently.

It is estimated that in England approximately one in 45 women will be exclusively homosexual, so an average general practice list of 2500 patients will have 20–30 women whose sexual interest is exclusively homosexual and more who have experimented (Hawton and Oppenheimer, 1993). Only a small proportion of these women will regard their homosexuality as a problem. All women are entitled to equality of health care. The narrative account of the health needs of the 'invisible minority' describes lesbian experiences of the health services and suggests how to improve health care for lesbian women.

Promoting continence is an integral part of health promotion. An insight into the aetiology and management of incontinence, as offered in the second part of the chapter, can influence the services offered within the general practice and improve the quality of life for many women.

Pre-menstrual syndrome (PMS), which affects many women, is poorly understood and inadequately managed. An appreciation of the underlying causes of PMS may assist the health professional to offer appropriate advice and support to sufferers.

The invisible minority: the health needs of lesbian women

There has been much debate in recent years concerning the health care needs of lesbians. However, in health arenas, this focus has shifted dramatically since the subject of female homosexuality was first identified. To understand fully the influences affecting the health of lesbians, it is essential to examine the historical context of lesbians within the health care system. Indeed, it was not until the turn of the century that the medical establishment focused their attention on the subject of female homosexuality.

Providing equitable health services demands that provision is culturally appropriate, sensitive and inclusive. Thus the purpose of this first part of the chapter is to demonstrate approaches that health providers may incorporate into their practice, creating safe inclusive health care for their lesbian clients.

Accessible, equitable and appropriately sensitive care relies on a deconstruction of the notion of a lesbian as a particular sort of woman who has specific health needs related to her sexuality. Lesbians are as similar, and as different, as all women, but socially constructed concepts of lesbianism entail common experiences that affect lesbians' use of and treatment by the health services.

Much has been written describing a reliance on the need to construct 'the other', the effect of which is increasingly to validate the lives of dominant groups in society and misconstrue and diminish the lives of those perceived to be different. What we have is women who, as a result of their life experiences, become the 'other'. It is hoped that many such myths can be dispelled through exploring the common issues in lesbian life experience.

Historical context

Research into the nature of female homosexuality was rare until the 1920s, before which biomedical science strove to classify and label every human condition, ignoring female homosexuality. Lesbians became the 'invisible women' of the twentieth century. Freud's (1920) publication of a book that included a chapter on women and homosexuality led to a change of focus, and a hunt ensued for the characteristics of those who suffered from it and for how it could be 'cured' (Haldeman, 1994).

The inclusion of homosexuality in the 'Diagnostic and Statistical Manual of Psychiatric Disorders' (DSM) created a fraught relationship between lesbians and health care providers. Visibility for lesbians relied solely upon their sexuality being placed clearly within the sickness paradigm, which led theorists to search for a cause, a treatment and a cure for this phenomenon (Haldeman, 1994). It was not until the 1950s, when Kinsey published the findings of his survey, that female homosexuality was recognized as a natural expression of human sexuality. This alteration in attitudes led ultimately to the removal of homosexuality from the DSM in 1973.

Unfortunately, this historical context left a damaging legacy whereby lesbians have been found to fear disclosure, rejection and exposure in health care environments and thus remain silent about their lives, their partners and their health concerns (Stevens, 1992; Hitchcock and Wilson, 1992). As a result, health providers are often found to perceive homosexuality as a problem reflecting the attitudes of some sections of the wider community.

Defining the population

The defining factor in lesbianism is relationships with women, but the nature of these relationships, and whether the individual is having relationships with women exclusively, varies enormously. Some lesbians have occasional emotional or sexual relationships with men, or have had very significant relationships with men before coming out. Others in the same position may prefer to define themselves as bisexual.

The variety of relationships is as diverse as that in the heterosexual community. Myths abound – the butch–femme dichotomy, predatory lesbians picking off heterosexual women – but they have no value as patterns, being only occasional occurrences that add to the variety of the whole. Same-sex relationships may have a much greater chance of the egalitarianism for which we all strive.

In discussing the health needs of lesbians, it is important to be broadly inclusive in defining the population. Lesbians are firstly women, women who are as diverse as the population at large, crossing every economic, racial, religious, age and ethnic boundary. One common feature of this group of women is their experience of stigmatization and marginalization, which can in turn lead to diminished access to appropriate health care (Simkin, 1991).

Self-disclosure

There are no rules, no guidelines to follow. People can become aware of their homosexuality at any time. With the realization invariably comes a painful internal struggle as people tussle with their feelings and following the social 'norm' to be heterosexual that has always been expected of them – that they have expected of themselves. The struggle often happens entirely alone, with little in the way of role models to follow and no one whom the individual feels she can trust sufficiently to open up to.

For many, information about sexuality is not accessible – learning about sexuality is a minefield of rumour, gossip and misinformation. Loneliness, depression and related disorders (anorexia nervosa) can ensue. The rate of suicide amongst young lesbian, gay and bisexual people is thought to be considerably higher than that amongst heterosexual youths (Savin Williams, 1994). Close family and friends may be aware that something is wrong but have little idea of the nature of the root of the problem; they simply do not want to know.

Concurrent with, or following, the self-disclosure of sexuality comes the traumatic task of coming out to other people: peers, colleagues, school friends, family ... . Coming out may be deliberate – a carefully thought-out process of testing the water – or can happen accidentally as other people begin to pick up signals that the individual is unaware she is giving out.

Coming out is a unique stress. The revelation of a significant part of an individual's make-up is seen by some people as socially unacceptable and by others as downright disgusting. Friends and family are seen as potential enemies to the self, leaving the individual isolated and alone.

Coming out is by no means a one-off event. Once the first crisis of self-disclosure has been overcome, a succession of crisis points in an individual's life follows as further people need to be told or find out, and the individual goes through a series of questioning of her own sexuality. Some lead a life failing to disclose their sexuality and significant aspects of their private lives to all but a very few, resulting in a constant fear of people finding out.

Whether sexuality should be revealed (or will be revealed accidentally) is a decision that has to be made when accessing services, particularly health-related services. This dilemma often leads to the individual avoiding the situation completely. Research by a women's sexual health project (SHADY, 1996) discovered that 29 per cent of lesbians and bisexual women had delayed using health services.

Coming out may be the first time individuals face homophobia. They will probably encounter this from school mates, colleagues, friends and family. As individuals, they may also have been homophobic themselves as part of their internal struggle for acceptance of themselves.

Facing homophobia is like facing a personal rejection, and this can come from those closest to the person. There is a huge spectrum of homophobia, and, as everyday stress affects each person differently, so the individual's ability to cope with it varies. From overt verbal or physical abuse to discrimination in the workplace, individuals can be stopped in their stride and prevented from living their lives as they would wish to.

Some individuals may come out fighting; others may withdraw into themselves becoming depressed and isolated. Others may need practical support such as legal advice or rehousing. Once faced with homophobia, individuals are far more likely to avoid other situations in which they have to reveal their homosexuality, including accessing services to help them in their current predicament.

Lesbians are as diverse as any other group of people, being from varied backgrounds and with vastly differing life experiences. These differences, coupled with anomalies in terminology, have important implications for service providers. Blanket approaches have limited applicability.

External pressures may impact on relationships. Family disapproval (or family exclusion from the knowledge of a relationship), for example, is not unusual. Even in accepting families, there can be problems simply in trying to accommodate a same-sex couple in usual family life. Invariably, although isolating, these external pressures come to the fore only where there exist, or they contribute to, problems in the relationship. A lesbian experiencing domestic violence from her partner, for instance, usually has no one to talk to, and no services available to help her through the situation.

Individuals may prefer to present as single rather than disclose their sexuality through revealing the gender of their partner (Hitchcock and Wilson, 1992). This self-negating act can be extremely demoralizing, especially before the wider family or in the workplace, where conversation often revolves around partners and home life.

Lesbian relationships, like any others, can of course bring great joy, stability and happiness. Children may further add to this joy. Individuals may bring children from previous relationships or may create their own family through adoption (where it is permitted) or donor insemination.

In 1987, Clause 28 (Creith, 1996) formalized a widespread disapproval of such families, which can act as a tremendous external pressure, but more pressing is the need for parents to protect their children from the homophobia and non-acceptance of their home lives that they will experience from school friends, teachers, grandparents and so on. Being 'different' is, in itself, an enormous pressure.

Health needs

The assumption is that current women's health care meets the needs of lesbian women. In fact, health services are generally not succeeding in catering for their needs. Equal access necessitates services being sensitive to the needs of all communities.

Recent research highlights very worrying trends in the uptake and experiences of health care by lesbians. For example, Stevens (1992) looked at 332 health care interactions involving lesbians across a wide range of health care facilities, providers and conditions. Seventy-seven per cent of these interactions were reported negatively. Research conducted by LesBeWell (1994) reported the following typical responses from lesbians discussing why they prefer not to go to their general practitioner:

> Their attitudes and language put up barriers for me.
> These days I will only go for medical treatment when it becomes very urgent.

Reasons given for being concerned about being a lesbian seeking treatment from a general practitioner included concerns about:

- confidentiality, both in terms of their homosexuality being revealed to potential employers seeking medical references, and in terms of their family;
- using the same practice or living and working in the same community as practice staff, where the individual's sexuality might be exposed through gossip or accidental disclosure.

Concerns were also voiced that lesbians would receive second-rate treatment if their sexuality were revealed in the practice. The following were typical reasons for not wanting to come out to primary health care providers:

> I'd be afraid they'd treat me differently.
> It would prejudice my treatment.

These beliefs often come from past negative experiences of coming out – to health providers or others – the fear of which is transferred to the current situation unless very positive indications are given that the same negative experiences will not recur. Primarily, however, the fear of revealing one's sexuality comes from a deep-seated understanding that homophobia is widespread:

> they would be shocked and horrified
> homophobia is prevalent in health services.

As homosexuality has until only very recently been seen as an illness or disorder in itself, there are also fears that individuals will still be seen as mentally ill and in need of a 'cure' for their sexuality.

The following section draws on the findings of research conducted by the health group LesBeWell; its purpose is to examine some of the difficulties experienced by lesbian patients and to offer suggestions for good practice.

Assumption of heterosexuality

> I feel that I can't be completely honest with her. She'll say something overtly heterosexual and I'll go back into the closet full speed.

The assumption of sexuality is pervasive in our society (Simkin, 1991). Signals highlighting the safety of their environment are easily detected by lesbians, and, although these signs if detected may be both subtle and inadvertent, lesbian patients may assume that the practice has not thought about people being gay and that its attitudes are negative. Many of the standard approaches to clients ask questions that have only heterosexual answers before any attempt is made to establish the patient's sexuality. Assessment forms usually query marital status, leaving a lesbian patient no option except to put 'single'. Including lesbian patients means substituting 'partner' as an option, providing the practice nurse with significant and relevant information and thus prompting more meaningful and insightful care (Hitchcock and Wilson, 1992).

By indicating this level of openness and inclusiveness, practice nurses are in a prime position to create the safe environment required for good rapport and the disclosure of other significant information necessary for accurate diagnosis and treatment.

> We'd lived together for 22 years, and she was still referred to as 'your friend'.

Involving a partner in a person's care is seen as good standard nursing practice. However, for many lesbians, this never becomes a reality. Involving a partner in care supports the goal of inclusive non-judgemental care. A thorough assessment of a patient includes discussion related to the patient's home and work life, her support networks and her relationship with her family.

Rushing to the conclusion of heterosexuality should be avoided unless explicitly confirmed, and this may be achieved by practice nurses reflecting upon and clarifying what may seem to be ambiguous information: 'Can I make a note of your partner's name?' or 'Do you have a partner? What is his or her name?' Such questions imply that the practice nurse has considered the diverse nature of human relationships and allow an appropriate next of kin to be recorded.

Confidentiality

> I wouldn't want such information on my records.
> My family see the same practice nurse.

Worries about confidentiality are commonplace yet, from a practitioner's perspective, may easily be overlooked. Many lesbian patients are apprehensive about disclosing personal information that may be recorded in their notes in what may be construed as a pejorative manner.

It is important to note that, should a breach of confidentiality occur, this is one matter about which a patient cannot complain without making matters much worse. In Britain, there is widespread discrimination against lesbians: in employment, in law and in the status of their relationships. Given this context, it is unsurprising that, for some lesbian clients, confidentiality becomes of paramount importance. Sharing of information should be done only with the explicit consent of the patient. Including sexual orientation in the medical notes can be done with consent and with a relevance to the nature of the problem. Once a lesbian is 'out', there is little a nurse can do to restore what may be a breach in confidentiality (see Chapter 1).

Sexual health

> I was told I didn't need smear tests – being gay.

For many women, the most probable initial interface with a practice nurse is the periodic smear test. Although lesbian health needs are primarily women's health needs, many lesbians are advised that they do not require cervical smear testing. As a result, many women present at longer intervals between smears or fail to attend at all.

Suggested risk factors for cervical screening appear to exclude lesbians from the screening criteria yet many lesbians have had earlier heterosexual activity, some are nulliparous, some have increased alcohol intakes and some have delayed child-bearing. In some situations, lesbians will present with these risk factors for both breast and cervical cancers (Council on Scientific Affairs, 1996). All women, whether heterosexually active or not, clearly require periodic cervical and breast screening. Additionally, where family relationships are either strained or have broken down, some lesbians may not have access to medical information that may indicate a family history of illness (Rankow, 1995).

The initial encounter with a practice nurse often includes two questions: 'Are you sexually active?' and 'What contraception are you using?' The responses to such questioning may create information that is both incomplete and inaccurate. In a similar way, the use of open-ended questions indicates the value placed on all life experiences. Asking instead, 'Do you need contraception?' or 'Are you sexually active with men, women or both?' supports the concept of not making judgements or assumptions about patients.

The lesbian family

The concept of a lesbian family is relatively new. With the introduction of Section 28 in 1987 (Creith, 1996), which sought to negate gay and lesbian partnerships as pretend family relationships, many lesbians have vehemently defended their rights to create families that do not conform to this rigid perspective. Therefore many lesbian families include children from past heterosexual relationships, through adoption and fostering, and of course through artificial insemination by donor (Dorsey Green, 1987). In some cases, lesbians may well present in a clinic seeking advice on insemination or even child care.

Lesbians considering parenting can be advised in much the same way as all women; however, attention to the role of the non-biological parent as an equal parent is essential. Due consideration may be given to the sensitivity of the legal status of lesbian relationships. At present, no automatic status is granted in gay and lesbian relationships; this includes the areas of inheritance, pensions, tenancy, immigration, taxation and parenting. It may be beneficial to recommend that, in such situations, an enduring power of attorney is created.

With these changes in family structure, a growing body of literature has examined the nature of lesbian families. Some theorists have

examined the parenting ability of lesbians, whilst others have investigated the mental health of children raised by lesbian parents. To
summarize, most studies concur that there is little difference between
this group and their heterosexual counterparts (Dorsey Green,
1987). In some cases, lesbian mothers may actually be more child
orientated and motivated. The assumptions made in many custody
cases of a weak parenting ability amongst lesbian mothers clearly
cannot be substantiated. Similarly, there is no evidence to suggest
that children raised in lesbian families experience greater levels of
stress. In contrast, many children have been found to be more
creative, more aware of their feelings and more relaxed.

Mental health

I wouldn't want them to think I was mentally ill.

Studies have attempted to counteract negative images with less
stereotypical ones, creating more positive and balanced perspectives.
Early studies suggest that, far from being bad for one's emotional
health, being lesbian can have positive effects upon it: in general,
lesbians were found to be more independent, more resilient, more
self-sufficient and more composed. Other studies found lesbians to
be better adjusted in some respects than women generally, and often
to achieve better job satisfaction (Hopkins, 1969; Siegelman, 1972).

Some studies have suggested that, amongst some health workers,
there is an assumption that sexual orientation is automatically linked
with mental distress. Lesbians do have unique concerns, which relate
to life in a homophobic world, but psychological illness is no more
common than in the wider population (Rankow, 1995). Some
women have been victims of homophobic incidents, whether these
be rejection from family and friends, verbal or physical attack, or a
denial of basic rights in housing, custody, employment (Bradford et
al., 1994; Savin Williams, 1994). Some women may indeed have
experienced this in health settings. Sensitivity to these realities is vital
if the practice nurse is to develop rapport with his or her lesbian
clients.

Internalized homophobia may also lead to low self-esteem and
isolation. This higher level of stress can sometimes lead some women
to self-destructive behaviours such as increased alcohol intake or
drug use. Young gay men and lesbians are thought to be at a considerably higher risk of suicide as a result of the prejudice and social
isolation they experience (Savin Williams, 1994). In all age groups,

lesbians may present in a health setting with stress-related physical health problems. By gentle and careful questioning, the practice nurse may be able to reveal underlying concerns and thus address physical problems appropriately.

Summary

Homophobia and heterosexism are not the fault of individual nurses but the legacy of their socialization. Health care that meets the needs of minority groups inevitably meets the needs of the mainstream.

Health professionals have a responsibility to explore their own biases, and work to eliminate attitudes that prevent the provision of, compassionate and inclusive health care (Eliason, 1992). Such health care should aim to be sensitive to the specific needs of all clients.

Some general practices are working proactively to reassure gay patients. Such initiatives include the display of relevant leaflets or posters. Gay and lesbian symbols, for example the Rainbow Freedom logo, can be displayed to indicate a practice's concern for this particular client group. Links with other agencies, including voluntary organizations, can be useful.

Health professionals who either ignore the needs of lesbians or advocate tolerance fail to address issues and experiences that are unique to lesbians and that require acknowledgment and understanding (Simkin, 1991). Education is the key to providing non-homophobic and non-heterosexist care. Nurses need to be knowledgeable about the needs of lesbian clients. Failing to address such attitudes may be seen as a breach of the nursing Code of Professional Conduct, in which nurses pledge to provide compassionate non-judgemental care to all.

Key points:

1. The assumption of heterosexuality must be addressed.
2. Confidentiality is paramount.
3. Any relationship must be validated.
4. The fear of labelling with a mental illness may deter a lesbian from seeking health care.

Promoting continence in general practice

Urinary incontinence is a devastating symptom with personal and social consequences often far more distressing than the root causes, which may be comparatively simple. At least 2 million people are known to be affected in the UK (Mandlestam, 1989), although for most people the condition is curable. Incontinence can be a symptom of many distinct underlying causes, so accurate diagnosis is crucial to successful treatment.

This section of the chapter will concentrate on female urinary incontinence. It aims to provide the reader with the practical and theoretical knowledge to assess the client through quality care, promoting clinical effectiveness and raising professional awareness. Early recognition of the problem and its underlying causes, together with planning and the provision of appropriate treatment, is fundamental in promoting continence.

Practice nurses are in a prime position to help sufferers through health education and increasing public awareness and acceptance of the condition. This should lead to an increased number of referrals to specialist continence advisers, which will improve the management of services and meet the needs of vulnerable groups such as younger disabled women, postnatal mothers and women with learning disabilities. This is not a definitive text but offers an insight into a complex subject area.

Definition of incontinence

Urinary incontinence is defined as an involuntary loss of urine that occurs more than twice a month and is a social or hygiene problem (Thomas et al., 1980).

Most continent people need to void less than once a night, and they can consciously control when and where micturition takes place. The severity of symptoms of incontinence varies between individuals: some may leak only a small amount occasionally, whilst others experience an almost continuous leakage (Norton, 1988).

Incontinence is not to do with the loss of control but with its location and timing. Continence depends very much on society's rules and acceptability of the place for voiding. Those who cannot, or do not, abide by these rules are thereby defined as 'incontinent'. Continence is voiding only in a socially acceptable place, whilst incontinence is voiding in the 'wrong' place.

The emphasis is placed on incontinence because it is either the symptom of a bladder dysfunction, the existence of factors rendering the person unable to cope with the bladder function, or the inability to learn bladder control by day and/or by night, or a combination of these factors. However, there is much that can be done if the underlying causes can be identified. Table 6.1 (pp 188–9) classifies systems for voiding dysfunction.

Incontinence can affect men and women of all ages and is independent of social class and ethnic origin. Women are more likely to experience problems than men of a similar age. Other groups of people at risk include children, people with learning and physical disabilities, those in residential care and older people.

Although the incidence increases with age, usually as a result of other pathology, incontinence must not be accepted as inevitable or incurable, although many suffer in silence rather than endure the stigma of incontinence (Norton, 1988). Many people believe incontinence to be a normal process of ageing, which obviously plays a major part in sufferers not seeking professional help (DoH, 1977).

Prevalence

Urinary incontinence is a subject that many people find difficult to discuss, although nurses are becoming more aware of continence issues. The figures shown in Box 6.1 suggest that at least 3 million people in the UK are regularly incontinent. In an average health district of approximately 250 000 people, 11 000 will be incontinent of urine (Millard, 1992). Of these, 77 per cent will be unknown to the health and social services (Cleave, 1991). About 25 per cent of women are severely incontinent (Thomas et al., 1980). Sufferers are inhibited from speaking out because of their feelings of guilt, shame, embarrassment and fear.

Box 6.1: Prevalence of urinary incontinence (Thomas et al. 1980)

- 1 in 4 women and 1 in 10 men suffer at some time in their lives
- 5% of the population experience urinary incontinence twice a month or more.

Types of incontinence

The following information forms the baseline from which further management is decided. Incontinence manifests as five different types, labelled I, II, III, IV and V.

Type I: Passive incontinence

The bladder fills and empties without sensation and unconsciously passes quantities of urine intermittently. This type of incontinence is invariably associated with major neurological disorders, disease, defect or injury to the brain or spinal cord.

Table 6.1: Classification systems for voiding dysfunction

Problem	Symptoms	Usual cause	Aggravation factors	Check for	Treatment	Medication
Genuine stress Stimulants	Coughing Sneezing Bending Exercise Lifting	Incompetent urethral sphincter Post-partum Menopause Prolapse Weight loss	Obesity Chronic cough Faecal impaction	Atrophic changes	Pelvic floor exercises Cones Pessaries Electrotherapy Treat cough	Oestrogen Alpha-stimulants Oestrogen replacement
Urge Anticholinergics	Urgency Frequency Nocturia	Unstable bladder (detrusor instability) Post surgical	UTI Anxiety Mobility difficulties Caffeine Alcohol Low fluid intake	UTI Neuropathy: over-flow obstruction	Bladder training Drug therapy Alternative therapy	(e.g. Oxybutynin, Imipramine, Propantheline) Oestrogen replace-ment if atrophic Extreme cases – surgery
Mixed age stress	May mimic pure stress, urge or mixed	Unstable bladder and sphincter incontinence	Obesity Chronic cough UTI Anxiety Low fluid intake	UTI Urodynamics	Bladder training Pelvic floor exercises Electrotherapy	Alpha-simulants Oestrogen replacement Anticholinergics; (surgery with caution unless instability)

(contd)

Table 6.1: (contd)

Problem	Symptoms	Usual cause	Aggravation factors	Check for	Treatment	Medication
Overflow obstruction	Passive dribble urgency Frequency Physical exertion	Overflow obstruction Hypotonic bladder Detrusor–sphincter dysynergia	Anticholinergics UTI	UTI Prostatic enlargement Faecal impaction Diabetes Neuropathy	Intermittent self-catheterization Avoid indwelling catheter when possible Clear faecal impaction Surgery to remove any obstruction	Treat UTI Prostate 5-alpha-reductase inhibitors
Functional severe intractable	Inability to reach toilet	Poor mobility Confusion, Dementia Lack of motivation Disabling environment	Sedation UTI Attitude of carers Diuretics	Faecal impaction UTI Mobility Dexterity Ability to use toilet	Improve environment Support carers Motivate Pads, appliances, catheters	Avoid medication Surgery not appropriate
Nocturnal enuresis	Wet bed when asleep (child/adult)	Idiopathic Familial Detrusor instability	Anxiety/stress Parental reaction Alcohol	UTI Congenital abnormalities	Enuresis alarm Star chart Bladder training	Antidiuretic hormone (desmopressin) Anticholinergics (oxybutynin imipramine) Surgery is rare

UTI = urinary tract infection

Type II: Dribble or overflow incontinence

The bladder is rarely or never contracted to expel urine, but a constant trickle escapes so that the patient is wet nearly all the time. This is accompanied by a significant reduction in bladder size and an increase in bladder neck tone (Bell et al., 1997) associated with disease, defect or injury to the brain or spinal cord, partial obstruction of the bladder outlet or drug therapy.

Type III: Stress/gynaecology incontinence

The International Continence Society defines stress incontinence as 'the involuntary loss of urine when the intravesical pressure exceeds the maximum urethral closure pressure in the absence of detrusor activity' (Colborn, 1994). This occurs during episodes of raised intra-abdominal pressure, such as coughing, sneezing and vigorous exercise.

Type III incontinence may follow childbirth (Cardozo et al., 1993) and gynaecological surgery (Donald, 1979).

Type IV: Reflex or sensory incontinence

The main characteristic of this type of incontinence is the occurrence of sudden floods of urine that take the patient completely by surprise. It comprises several categories:

- *Autonomic bladder:* the patient involuntarily passes small quantities of urine periodically.
- *Atonic bladder:* the patient's loss of awareness of distension of the bladder wall leads to the chronic retention of urine and the continuous leakage of an overflow.
- *Reflux bladder:* incomplete emptying of the bladder results in leakage and residual urine.
- *Uninhibited bladder:* the awareness of bladder distension is interpreted as an urgent need to pass urine and is followed very quickly by the contraction that causes the bladder to open.

Type V: Urge/frequency incontinence

The symptoms may appear very similar to those of types III and IV incontinence, or a combination of both. Before passing urine, the patient experiences the sensation of needing to micturate, but the onset of the sensation is sudden and very quickly changes to urgency.

This is followed almost immediately by irresistible contractions of the bladder.

This sequence of events can happen when the bladder is only partly full, sometimes only a few minutes after it has been emptied. It is associated with disease, defect or injury of the spinal column, disease of the bladder or urethra, drug therapy, emotional stress and physical disability.

Provocation occurs through coughing and vigorous exercise, laughing and caffeine and citrus fruit intake; it can result in the woman leaking urine before she reaches a toilet. In addition, she will commonly experience persistent frequency and nocturnal enuresis. Known as detrusor instability (or unstable bladder), this condition can be objectively demonstrated by urodynamic investigations.

It is important to distinguish between stress and urge incontinence since both can result in leakage after coughing. The diagnosis can be made following urodynamic investigations. However, mixed symptoms may occur, a common situation in post-menopausal women. Lowered oestrogen levels affect the urethral closure mechanism, which then becomes less effective, and are associated with bladder outlet incompetence because of weakness of the supporting pelvic floor muscles (Figure 6.1).

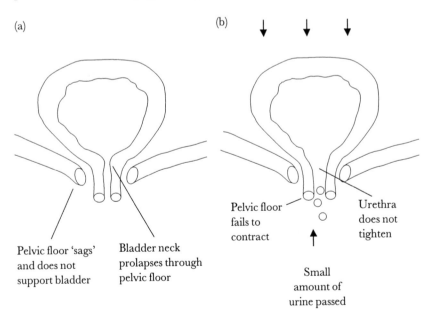

(a)

(b)

Pelvic floor fails to contract

Urethra does not tighten

Small amount of urine passed

Pelvic floor 'sags' and does not support bladder

Bladder neck prolapses through pelvic floor

Figure 6.1: (a) Illustrates stress incontinence caused by weakness of the pelvic floor muscles. (b) Coughing, laughing, running, etc. causes a rise in intra-abdominal pressure, which results in leakage of urine.

Pelvic floor

'Pelvic floor' is the term used to describe a group of muscles that form a 'hammock' sling from each side of the pubic bone to the sacrum and coccyx. If the muscles are overstretched during childbirth, the gap in the muscles around the urethra and vagina is widened, and the support to the bladder weakens. The most important part of the pelvic floor is the deepest layer of muscles, collectively called the levatores ani. Possible sources of damage to the pelvic floor include:

- childbirth;
- chronic constipation and straining at stool;
- surgery;
- radiotherapy;
- trauma.

It can be seen that incontinence is a complex issue, involving either the pelvic floor muscles, bladder instability or both. Correct assessment is therefore essential.

Assessing the problem

Assessment is the basis of appropriate continence advice. The aim of assessment is to identify the type of incontinence and alleviate the distress caused by the condition. A nurse who does not have the relevant ENB 978 qualification equivalent training, or who does not feel competent to address the problem, should refer the woman to a continence adviser for specialist advice (see Chapter 1).

Assessment is a key factor in individual care. Newton (1991) defined assessment as 'collecting information, reviewing it, identifying the patient's problems and prioritising the problems gained through observation, interview, examination, measurement and investigations as appropriate to the individual'.

The assessment must take into account the patient's comprehension of the problems and her ability to look after herself. This includes diet, fluid intake and environment (is there easy access to a toilet, for example?), medication and family history.

Verbal and non-verbal communication make a valuable contribution towards assessing physical, mental, social and environmental factors affecting the patient, some or all of which may be causal factors for incontinence. It is important to establish a relationship of trust through good communication skills to ensure that the consultation environment is free from disturbance (Brown, 1994). Confidentiality is paramount as the patient may not wish family members to know about the continence problems; the presence of another person may also inhibit a woman fully expressing herself.

The use of an examination checklist (Box 6.2), an examination (Box 6.3), investigations (Box 6.4) and referral pathways to promote continence (Fig 6.2) may be useful in identifying those suffering from incontinence.

The nurse is advised to follow written procedural guidelines, or protocols, to conduct a basic comprehensive assessment (see Chapter 2). Assessments may be more effective if carried out by a team that includes doctors, nurses and professionals allied to medicine. Where special investigations may be necessary to identify bladder dysfunction, the nurse must be the patient's advocate and refer, when neces-

---

Box 6.2: Continence assessment checklist (adapted from Smith & Nephew, 1992)

If the assessment checklist is used as a separate document from the patient's medical records, personal details must be recorded to identify the individual

Clinical and social issues that must be addressed in a comprehensive assessment include:

- presenting problem;
- patient's medical history, including obstetric history;
- patient's sexual history;
- patient's own and family continence history;
- patient's perception of the problem;
- the referring clinician's perception of the problem;
- urinary symptoms;
- bowel symptoms, including constipation and/or diarrhoea;
- voiding patterns;
- current medication;
- other clinical problems;
- social problems;
- dietary habits;
- fluid intake (should remain in the range 1500–2500 ml per day);
- mobility;
- dexterity;
- psychological state;
- social activities;
- personal relationship;
- home environment;
- types of aid and/or pad used and their effectiveness

Box 6.3: Continence assessment – examination

The type of examination required to identify urinary incontinence lies within the province of a registered nurse.

Observe the following:
- the clothes for severity of incontinence;
- incontinence aids;
- abdominal distension, which may be due to a full bladder or a pelvic tumour (e.g. ovarian cyst), or obesity;
- vaginal discharge;
- prolapse: rectocele, cystocele or uterine prolapse;
- atrophic vaginitis;
- condition of pelvic floor muscle;
- anal examination to observe the anal sphincter: if this is damaged, it may affect the urethral sphincter; may detect constipation

---

Box 6.4: Continence assessment – investigations

- Urinalysis/MSU
- Blood tests for urea and electrolytes, and full blood count
- Frequency/volume charting
- Rectal and vaginal examination
- Urodynamic tests, measuring pressure changes as they occur within the bladder and urethra during filling:
  - cystometry: measures pressure within the bladder;
  - urogram: intravenous pyelogram (IVP) to X-ray any part of the urinary tract
- Abdominal ultrasound and/or bladder scan to exclude a tumour
- Digital assessment to investigate pelvic floor function. This assesses the strength of the pelvic floor muscles, graded from 0 to 5, where 0 = no strength and 5 = strong

---

sary, to the GP or continence adviser. Some women will need to be referred to, and examined by, a gynaecologist, urologist, neurologist or physician before the cause of the incontinence can be confirmed and a treatment plan agreed.

The woman should be provided with a contact name and telephone number for access to the service, including the names and addresses of local or national support groups (see Useful addresses).

Activity 6.1: Liaise with colleagues and devise a protocol for continence assessment and management. This should include referral pathways.

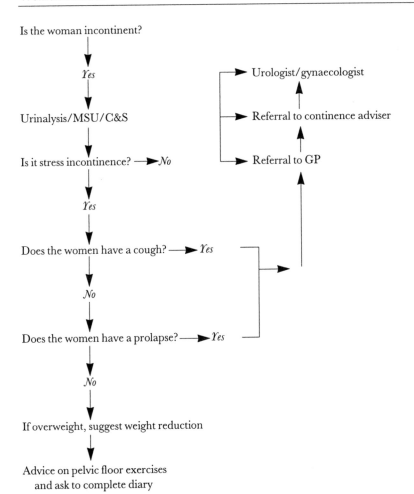

Figure 6.2: Referral pathways to promote continence. MSU = mid-stream urine; C&S = culture and sensitivity.

Multidisciplinary approach to continence management

For those women with urinary incontinence who seek help, their first point of contact is often the primary health care team. According to Duffin and Castleden (1986), over 50 per cent of patients who had informed someone about their incontinence had spoken to their general practitioner. All too often, the general practitioner simply referred the woman to the district nurse, feeling that incontinence and its management were her domain. Mathiason (1992) quotes from one general practitioner: 'a conspiracy of silence surrounds the problem'. Patients often do not come forward, and, when they do, doctors do not want to know.

To overcome negative responses, it is important to establish a multidisciplinary strategy for the promotion of urinary continence and the management of incontinence, and a comprehensive quality service that should be seen to embrace both primary and secondary care. It is essential that good liaison and working relationships exist in order to provide a seamless service to the local population in line with Department of Health guidelines (DoH, 1977). The team is likely to encompass the individuals described below.

General practitioners and practice nurses

General practitioners and practice nurses are usually the patient's starting point and often have the overall picture of their client's problems, having undertaken a physical assessment and investigations. They generally co-ordinate the efforts of all other team members in order to enable the appropriate management of incontinence (see Table 6.1 above).

Continence adviser

This specialist nurse provides advice, training and a specialist service on continence problems, investigations and the treatment of incontinence. He or she will usually make arrangments for continence aids if required.

Urologist/gynaecologist

Specialist investigations to diagnose a cause for incontinence, carried out by these physicians, are necessary for some women (see Box 6.4 above).

Physiotherapist

The physiotherapist will assess mobility and difficulties, and may be able to suggest an appropriate treatment.

Occupational therapist

The occupational therapist will assess functional ability and environmental factors, including manual dexerity and access to toilet facilities.

Psychologist

The implications of incontinence can be assessed by the psychologist.

Social worker

The social worker can play a key role in situations where the implications of incontinence fall outside the nurse's remit, for example where a mattress or bedding is ruined.

> **Activity 6.2: Identify the relevant multidisciplinary team for continence management in your general practice. Liaise with each member to identify the specific role of each health professional. This may vary between authorities.**

Promoting continence

During consultations, it is best to avoid using the word 'incontinence', as to many people this means a complete loss of control. Women may deny incontinence but admit to the 'occasional leak' or 'accident'. The flow chart in Figure 6.2 above demonstrates a referral pathway that will assist a management programme for promoting continence.

Following a comprehensive assessment, an individual plan of care must be formulated with the woman. This will include goals of care and a review date for follow-up assessment. The follow-up assessment is summarized in Box 6.5 but can be adapted to individual requirements.

Box 6.5: Follow-up assessment checklist

Name .... DOB...............

Assessment date...............

1. Are your symptoms improving, static, worsening?..

2. How often do leaks occur?...

3. How often are you doing your pelvic floor exercises?..

4. If you are not carrying out pelvic floor exercises, what is preventing you doing so?...

5. What level of distress does your problem cause you, on a scale of 1 to 10, 10 being most severe?

None   1   2   3   4   5   6   7   8   9   10   Maximum

The above assessment may help when collecting data towards an audit.

The first-line management for stress incontinence may be pelvic floor exercises (Box 6.6). The woman should notice an improvement with her symptoms after three months.

Box 6.6: Pelvic floor exercises

- To identify the pelvic floor, next time you are passing urine, try to stop in the middle of the stream The muscles you use to do this are called the pelvic floor muscles
- Like any muscle, the more they are exercised, the stronger they become
- Squeeze these muscles, count to 4 and relax the muscles. Repeat this exercise four times
- The exercises should be performed at least ten times a day, every day. The more frequently you exercise, the stronger the pelvic floor becomes and the quicker the improvement in urinary continence
- These exercises can be carried out at any time, so no one is aware you are doing them
- Pelvic floor exercises can be linked with any hourly event of the day, such as the news bulletin on the radio or when you have a drink
- Note: do not regularly do pelvic floor exercises while passing urine. However, you can try this once a week to check the progress of urinary continence
- An improvement should be noticed after 3 months

Progress should be reviewed in 6 weeks and a further appointment arranged as necessary

---

A voiding diary is a valuable tool in management. It can be used to document information about patterns of urinary elimination both during initial assessment and when evaluating the effectiveness of a bladder management programme. The diary serves several purposes, including the assessment of diurnal and nocturnal voiding, and incontinence patterns. More detailed diaries may be used to document behavioural or environmental factors that precipitate or alleviate leakage. The selection of a voiding diary is guided by the type of information sought, the motivation and knowledge of the person completing the diary, and the type or types of voiding being documented.

An effective diary may be kept over 4–7 days for detailed data. When a voiding diary is kept for too long, the individual may become bored or frustrated and the accuracy of data is often reduced. An example of a voiding diary is illustrated in Figure 6.3.

The nurse may wish a patient to be referred to an appropriate consultant. This will usually follow general practitioner intervention, although nurse practitioners have the advantage of referring directly

Date.................... Name.................... DOB....................

Add in 1st column the amount of fluid by the cup (e.g. 1 cup)
Tick in 2nd column each time urine is passed.
Tick in 3rd column each time you are wet.

TIME	MON			TUES			WED			THUR			FRI			SAT			SUN		
	fluid intake	urine passed	urine leaked	fluid intake	urine passed	urine leaked	fluid intake	urine passed	urine leaked	fluid intake	urine passed	urine leaked	fluid intake	urine passed	urine leaked	fluid intake	urine passed	urine leaked	fluid intake	urine passed	urine leaked

Figure 6.3: Voiding diary.

to hospital services. There is usually a direct referral route to specialist physiotherapy, continence and district nurse services. The triggers
for referral, summarized in Box 6.7, must be clearly stated in the
clinical practice treatment protocol. The case-study below demonstrates an assessment and treatment plan in action.

Box 6.7: Specialist referral (adapted from Smith & Nephew, 1992)

Triggers that prompt further referral to an appropriate specialist include:

- no improvement within 3 months of implementing the care plan, for example pelvic floor exercises, voiding diary, drug therapy or physiotherapy;
- a need for specialist tests: urodynamic investigations, bladder or vaginal
  scan;
- problems with incontinence products and equipment;
- recurrent medical problems

Case-study 6.1

Mrs B, a 62-year-old lady, presented in general practice with continence problems.

Patient's perception of the problem: Always going to the toilet and sometimes not getting there in time. Having to get up at least three times a
night.

Obstetric history: Three children all under 8 lb 5 oz, no forceps, one
tear with suturing of the perineum and internal sutures.

Medical history: Irritable bowel for 6 years, very anxious lady, a
worrier, prone to coughs and colds. Hormone replacement therapy for
4 years.

Surgical history: Abdominal hysterectomy 9 years ago. Fusion of L3
and L4 vertebrae 5 years ago. Still suffering back pain from muscle
spasm, for which she takes analgesics.

Assessment: Pelvic floor muscle grade 3 (moderate). Hold pelvic floor
muscle for 5 seconds, repetition of eight quick contractions five times.

Investigations: Urinalysis NAD; referred for urodynamic investigations, which confirmed detrusor instability.

Treatment implemented: Bladder re-education using frequency/
volume of urine charting for 1 week (see Figure 6.3). Pelvic floor exercises to strengthen pelvic floor muscles.

Instructions provided: Pelvic floor exercises are to help to control the
urge to go to the toilet so that the feeling fades away and the woman
holds on for another 15 minutes.

Assessed 4 weeks later: In Mrs B's opinion, still not much progress.
However, on observing the symptoms over the past 2 weeks, she
realized that the nocturia had reduced to twice a night and some-

times only once. Urodynamic results discussed and anticholinergic tablets prescribed, one to be taken twice daily, to help the urgency. Mrs B referred to the continence adviser for monitoring.

Two months later: Daytime frequency improved to seven times a day and once at night. As a side effect of drug treatment was a dry mouth, anticholinergic treatment reduced to each morning and alternate evenings. Mrs B beginning to feel better and had learned to control her urgency.

One month later: Daytime frequency down to six times a day, and a longer urine volume being voided. Occasional nocturia. Mrs B had developed nightmares. Further reduction in anticholinergic to alternate mornings only; nightmares stopped. Mrs B remained on this dose of medication to maintain and improve bladder control. A 6-monthly post-voiding residual urine measurement arranged.

Six months later: Mrs B discharged from the continence clinic a much happier lady, now in control of her bladder. The 6-monthly assessment of residual urine allowed her contact and support.

Summary: Complex issues sensitively managed, and referral for specialist advice made as appropriate.

> **Activity 6.3: Begin an audit of continence management in your practice. You may wish to determine the effectiveness of pelvic floor exercises, the number of women helped by anticholinergic therapy or how many women required surgery to manage their incontinence. You may need to reassess your protocol following this audit.**

Summary

The opportunity for screening urinary incontinence should be incorporated into routine practice. Well-women, cervical screening, family planning and disease management assessment clinics, as well as postnatal sessions, are ideal opportunities to enquire about urinary problems. These problems may also be identified during any other consultation, particularly when health professionals have a high level of awareness.

It must be recognized that some women prefer to wait to see how a minor continence problem progresses. These women must be reassured that they can return for review and referral at any time.

Practice nurses are in a privileged position. They have access to intimate information and are trusted and respected for their advice. Women must be encouraged to seek help and not to tolerate incontinence as a fact of life. Promoting continence through appropriate and sensitive intervention can improve the quality of life for many women.

Key points:

1. Seventy-seven per cent of sufferers are unknown to the health or social services.
2. Most cases of incontinence can be cured.
3. The expertise of a multidisciplinary team should be applied.
4. Incontinence is not an inevitable part of ageing.

Pre-menstrual syndrome

Pre-menstrual syndrome (PMS) is an increasingly topical and controversial subject that is also confusing because, despite attention in the medical journals, its existence is still disputed. This section will provide the reader with an insight into the complexity of PMS, a common condition with which women present to both the general practitioner and the gynaecologist. The first step in helping women with PMS is for health professionals to recognize the importance of the disorder and to distinguish true PMS from the milder and more common psychological symptoms or even psychiatric disorders. The latter have symptoms unrelated to the ovarian endocrine cycle. Failure to make these two distinctions has led to inappropriate and ineffective treatment (O'Brien, 1993).

Although its cause remains either uncertain or multifactorial, PMS includes a wide range of physical, psychological and behavioural symptoms. The following text addresses the issues surrounding PMS in order to enable nurses to recognize the syndrome and offer appropriate support and management to sufferers.

Definition

Many doctors do not believe that there is such a condition and consequently fail to recognize and treat PMS. To compound the situation, there is no universally accepted definition (Andrews, 1994). However, Taylor (1983) has cited the Royal College of Obstetricians and Gynaecologists working party, which, in 1993, identified that 'a woman can be said to be suffering from PMS if she complains of regularly recurring psychological or somatic symptoms, or both, which occur regularly in the same phase of the menstrual cycle followed by a symptom-free period of less than seven days'.

Menstrual distress refers to symptoms present through the menstrual cycle and exacerbated pre-menstrually (Mascarenas, 1990).

Pre-menstrual symptoms were recognized by the medical profession in 1931. An American gynaecologist, Robert Frank, used the term 'pre-menstrual syndrome' to describe the problem associated with the normal experiences of menstruation (Andrews, 1994). This was possibly because, in the early part of the century, a woman's fertile years were fewer in number: menarche was uncommon before the age of 14 or 15, and menopause occurred at 35–40 years of age. Most women spent their intervening years either pregnant or lactating, so the menstrual cycle played a less dominant part in their lives (Mascarenas, 1990).

A cross-cultural study of menstruation found that the majority of women in all the cultures investigated reported physical discomfort, and that negative mood changes were widely experienced (Woods et al., 1992).

Aetiology

It is difficult to assess how common PMS symptoms are as so many women do not discuss their symptoms. However, surveys suggest that about 85 per cent of women have experienced PMS symptoms (Mascarenas, 1990), although Glynn (1993) has found disagreement between contemporary researchers. Although the cause of PMS remains either uncertain or multifactoral, nutritional and lifestyle factors are now thought to be a consideration, particularly as hormonal and pharmacological preparations have failed as broadly successful treatments (Stewart et al., 1992).

The cause of PMS symptoms are still unclear, although two areas are considered by some clinicians to be contributory:

- hormone imbalance owing to inadequate levels of progesterone;
- dietary imbalance because of a lack of certain vitamins, magnesium and zinc, and a deficiency of essential fatty acids.

The medical model suggests that PMS is linked to abdominal changes. One factor recognized by Taylor (1983) and Henshaw and Smith (1993) was the deficiency of ovarian progesterone secretion in the luteal phase of the menstrual cycle.

The current consensus is that normal ovarian function, rather than hormone imbalance, is the cyclical trigger for biomedical events with the central nervous system and other target tissues. This view is supported by O'Brien (1993), who found that hormonal abnormalities did not occur with any great regularity. There has been a growing recognition that oestrogen and progesterone directly affect nerve cell functioning and thus have profound influences on behaviour, mood and the processing of sensory information (Sutherland, 1990).

Symptoms

Pre-menstrual distress describes a variety of symptoms recurring in the same phase of the menstrual cycle. This is usually 2–7 days before menstruation and is relieved by the onset of menses. It appears to be more common in women over the age of 30 and is often precipitated by childbirth (Kleijnen et al., 1990). Other predisposing factors include stressful or emotional life events such as bereavement or divorce, or psychiatric disorders (Glynn, 1993). Such symptoms may also be associated with the oral contraceptive pill (Henshaw and Smith, 1993).

Kleijnen et al. (1990) suggest that the elevated levels of oestrogen found in women suffering from PMS may result from the body's own inability, because of vitamin deficiency, to break down the oestrogen for excretion. Oestrogen production is also dramatically influenced when body weight falls below or exceeds 20 per cent of ideal body weight, as oestrogen levels fall (Stewart et al., 1992).

Recent research shows that pre-menstrual symptoms often persist in women on hormone replacement therapy that includes progesterone (Hickerton, 1994), and in women who have had a hysterectomy with conservation of their ovaries, as it appears to be cyclical progestogen that causes most of the problems, although symptoms are abolished by hysterectomy and bilateral oopherectomy (Henshaw and Smith, 1993). Research has also shown that women given oestrogen therapy after hysterectomy and oopherectomy do not develop PMS symptoms (O'Brien, 1993). PMS symptoms are unknown in post-menopausal women (Mascarenas, 1990).

PMS has previously received very little attention from doctors, but there has in recent years been an upsurge of interest, numerous books and articles in women's magazines having been written on the subject. A survey by the Womens Nutritional Advisory Service highlighted the association between increased caffeine intake, cigarette smoking, low exercise levels and increased pre-menstrual symptoms (Stewart et al., 1992).

Dalton (1980) describes how three women were acquitted of their crimes of manslaughter, arson and assault, having pleaded mitigation with diminished responsibility because of pre-menstrual symptoms. Dalton's extensive description of individual case-studies showed that women who sought help complained of multiple symptoms during the 12 days preceding menstruation.

Many of the presenting symptoms described in PMS are listed in Table 6.2, and the systemic changes are given in Table 6.3. Depending on the severity of symptoms, a woman's home, work and social life can be severely affected and her quality of life reduced.

Table 6.2: Pre-menstrual symptoms (adapted from Moos, 1968)

Physical	
Water retention	Weight gain
	Abdominal bloating
	Peripheral oedema
Pain	Pelvic pain
	Breast tenderness
	Headache/migraine
	Abdominal pain
	Muscle stiffness
	General aches and pains
General	Exacerbation of epilepsy, asthma, rhinitis, urticaria and skin conditions
	Change in bowel habit/constipation/ diarrhoea
	Tinnitus
	Numbness and tingling
	Palpitations
Psychological	
Concentration	Depression
	Emotional instability
	Fatigue
	Clumsiness or poor co-ordination
	Insomnia
	Irritability
	Decrease/increase in libido
	Memory impairment
	Concentration difficulty
	Prone to accidents
	Confusion
	Difficulty making decisions
	Agoraphobia/claustrophobia
	Suicidal feelings
	Mood swings
	Panic attacks
Behavioural	Personality changes, e.g. mood swings, irritability and restlessness
	Lowered work performance
	Absenteeism from work or school
	Avoidance of social activities
	Loss of efficiency
	Need for more or less sleep
	Food cravings for sweets and carbohydrates

(contd)

Table 6.2: (contd)

Negative effects	Depression
	Tension
	Crying spells
	Loneliness
	Anxiety
Arousal	Feeling affectionate
	Orderliness
	Excitement
	Feeling of well-being
	Bursts of energy/activity
Autonomic reaction	Cold sweats/hot flushes
	Feeling dizzy or faint
	Nausea or vomiting

Table 6.3: Systemic changes during the menstrual cycle

Item	Nature of change
Temperature	Decreases at time of ovulation, then sharp rise to a plateau
Blood pressure	Arterial pressure lower mid-cycle
Respiration	Increased ventilation of lung with decreased arterial carbon dioxide tension in the luteal phase
Weight	Some women gain in the pre-menstrual period
Carbohydrate metabolism	Tolerance to glucose is less (fasting blood sugar level is higher) during menstruation
Cholesterol	Total serum cholesterol rises following menstruation
Thyroid	Pre-menstrual rise in basal metabolic rate during menstruation
Skin	Darkening of skin pre-menstrually is related to increased sensitivity to ultraviolet light; increased sebaceous gland activity pre-menstrually; fewer active sweat glands during luteal phase
Breast	Pre-menstrual hyperaemia and increased breast size

The character and intensity of the symptoms may vary from woman to woman and in different cycles. One woman may be able to identify only one or two symptoms in a mild form in a particular cycle, whilst women who experience more severe effects may experience several symptoms.

In trying to establish a cause for PMS, there are a number of hypotheses, including:

- the involvement of the ovarian hormones oestradiol and progesterone;
- disturbed function of the central mechanisms influencing the menstrual cycle;
- the actions of prolactin or androgens;
- a deficient or excessive production of prostaglandins or endorphins;
- hypoglycaemia;
- low magnesium levels;
- numerous psychological and social factors.

The symptoms vary so widely between individuals and even between cycles for an individual that it is likely that different aetiological factors apply to different women.

Diagnosis

Because of the widespread publicity given to PMS by the lay press and the media in recent years, the diagnosis of PMS is often made by women themselves. Women go to their physicians or psychotherapists saying, 'I have PMS.' The doctor then evaluates whether the woman does indeed experience cyclical symptoms, their severity and whether they are related to other disorders such as depression, dysmenorrhoea, an endocrine disturbance or another cause.

However, a woman's past experience with doctors will influence her future decisions on the need for medical advice. In a study of women who menstruated, Scrambler and Scrambler (1985) identified that a third of their sample had consulted their general practitioner with respect to menstrual distress and discomfort. The remainder of the sample did not seek medical help because they felt disillusioned with their doctors. Many women found that their doctors were unresponsive, unsympathetic and unable to help. Most of the doctors were male, which made seeking help more difficult. It is to be hoped that this scenario will become less common with the increasing number of women doctors in general practice. The fulfilment of a patient's expectations and requirements when seeking help for pre-menstrual symptoms may depend upon the effectiveness of communication between the health professional and the patient.

It has also been suggested that PMS may result from negative attitudes acquired during socialization. PMS researchers and clinicians acknowledge that the variability of PMS can in fact be attributed to its conceptualization. This negative aspect of socialization may hinder the process and affect diagnosis. Studies have suggested that doctors may record the psychological and emotional problems experienced by many women during the pre-menstrual phase and dismiss them as psychosomatic (Bernstein and Kane, 1981). O'Brien (1993) states how PMS has been dismissed by many doctors because their experiences have been limited to observations of their own cycles or those of their wives or female colleagues. It is essential for doctors to recognize the condition in order for women to receive help and support.

Diagnosis can be made on the basis of history as there are no specific laboratory tests to diagnose PMS. If symptoms recur cyclically and are relieved by the start or cessation of menses, diagnosis can be made if the absence of other pathophysiological and psychological disorders has been determined (Mascarenas, 1990). However, there is little evidence that menstrual distress alone will drive a normal individual to desperate behaviour. Psychiatric referral is necessary for only a small number of sufferers (Sampson, 1984).

When making a differential diagnosis, physical and psychological factors frequently produce a similar or an identifiable pattern. Care needs to be exercised when relying on the self-reporting of symptoms.

A useful means of establishing whether PMS is present is through the use of a personal diary (Figure 6.4). This involves completing a daily calendar over a period of three months before any treatment is commenced. Symptoms are noted using a coding system chart, preferably at the same time each day, in order to identify a PMS pattern of symptoms.

To clarify the diagnosis in difficult cases, a formal psychiatric evaluation, including detailed analysis, a structured internal and an objective questionnaire, may help to determine into which category the woman fits (O'Brien, 1987). It may help the reader to discuss a difficult case with a mental health nurse before making a formal referral.

Activity 6.4: You may like to do an informal survey of your female colleagues and friends to identify the number who have unmanaged PMS symptoms. List the most commonly reported symptoms and the most common home management remedies. This may help you to identify sufferers and offer 'tried and tested' remedies.

Code	Symptom
T	Tension
I	Irritability
D	Depression
A	Anxiety
F	Fatigue
DC	Difficulty with concentation
AC	Abdominal cramps
H	Headache
BA	Backache
MS	Muscle spasm
BT	Breast tenderness
WG	Weight gain
S	Swelling of joints (fingers and ankles)
B	Bloating
AH	Abdominal heaviness

The woman is asked to complete a diary using the symptom code

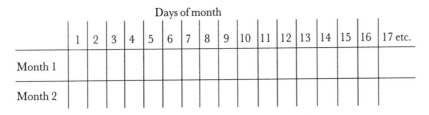

Figure 6.4: Example of a menstrual diary.

Management

The evidence suggests that PMS is an endocrine problem of multiple and complex aetiology, with different women experiencing different forms of endocrine upset (Gould, 1990). It therefore seems unlikely that a single treatment regime will prove 100 per cent effective for all.

PMS is still incompletely understood, although there are many treatments that have been tried. Box 6.8 illustrates the wide variety of prescribed drugs and hormone preparations that are used to relieve symptoms, with varying degrees of popularity and success.

Dalton's case-studies support hormone therapy for women who exhibit antisocial behaviour; their behaviour returned to normal following treatment with progesterone (Dalton, 1980).

Figure 6.5 (see p. 211) illustrates an example of pathways to effective treatment. Women with psychological pre-menstrual changes will benefit from counselling and reassurance, and those with non-cyclical psychiatric problems should be helped by the early identification of their problems with appropriate referral (O'Brien, 1993).

Box 6.8: Medical treatment options for PMS

- Counselling
- Vitamin B6 (pyridoxine)/vitamin E/multivitamins
- Magnesium
- Evening primrose oil (Efamast)
- Diuretics
- Gonadotrophin releasing hormone (Danazol)
- Combined oral contraceptive pill
- Oestradiol patches, implants
- Progestogen (Norethisterone, Primolut N)
- Progesterone (Cyclogest)
- Dydrogesterone (Duphaston)
- Tranquillizers and antidepressants
- Surgery

Case-studies 6.2 and 6.3 demonstrate how treatment can be successful if both the doctor and the woman are prepared to try different remedies. The practice nurse will usually follow a holistic approach to health, although she may be required to encourage compliance with treatment.

Case-study 6.2

Mrs W was a 36-year-old housewife and mother of three children. She complained of symptoms clearly suggesting the pre-menstrual syndrome for 10–14 days before each period, which she had experienced for the past four years. Her menstrual cycle was 39 days. Mrs W's main complaints were of severe breast tendernesss, lethargy, mood swings (depression and irritability), troublesome bloating and bad co-ordination in the 14 days prior to the onset of menses.

Management: Blood tests to assess prolactin and oestradiol levels showed no abnormality. Mrs W had been treating herself for the past 12 months with evening primrose oil and multivitamins, with very little relief. Dietary and lifestyle changes were addressed, and observation over a period of three months with the aid of a symptom diary highlighted the above symptoms.

Mrs W was referred to her GP, who prescribed progesterone suppositories, pyridoxine and diuretics, with very little relief. Four capsules of Efamast (Gamolenic acid) were prescribed twice daily, which resulted in an improvement in mood and some reduction in swelling and breast discomfort. This was mainatined during patient follow-up three months later. Mrs W was maintained on a lower dose of two capsules of Efamast daily, which controlled her PMS symptoms.

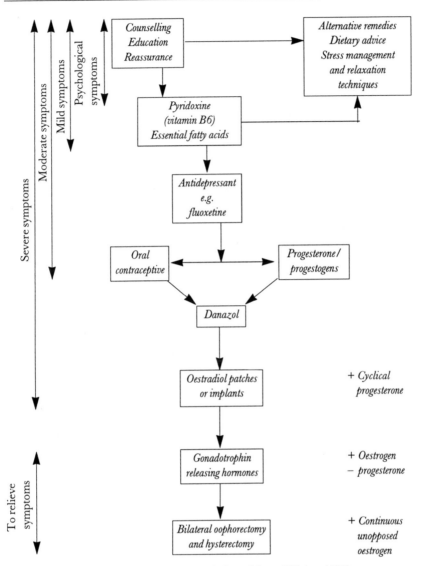

Figure 6.5: Pathways to effective treatment (adapted from O'Brien, 1993).

Case-study 6.3

Miss K was a 28-year-old nulliparous secretary, who had complained of pre-menstrual symptoms for the past five years. Her symptoms were similar to Mrs W's (see Case-study 6.2).

Management: Blood tests showed normal oestradiol and prolactin levels. Miss K had previously been treated with tranquilisers and diuretics, with no benefit. On review, the symptom diary chart recorded over a period of three months highlighted breast discomfort, mood swings and swelling. She was prescribed three capsules of Efamast and one tablet of pyridoxine twice daily. In addition, Miss K was given educational support, dietary advice and stress management techniques. This management combination resulted in complete symptom relief.

The role of the practice nurse

Patients often want to discuss treatments for PMS, many of which can be obtained without prescription, that they have read about in magazines (Box 6.9).

Practice nurses are in a prime position to fulfil a valuable function in primary care for those women who seek help for health-related problems such as PMS. Women may be more willing to seek help from practice nurses than from doctors as most nurses are female. Nurses may identify women with PMS during routine well-woman or general health checks, either through appropriate and sensitive questioning, or through an observation of change of behaviour.

Careful evaluation of symptoms and psychological status (see Table 6.2) must be assessed before individual treatment programmes are devised. Those identified as having psychological pre-menstrual changes will initially require counselling, although most will find some relief in being able to talk to an empathetic listener. Stress management, relaxation, dietary recommendations, alternative therapies and psychotherapy support may help some women to cope with their symptoms (Box 6.9).

Box 6.9: Treatments for PMS available without a prescription

- Dietary advice
- Exercise programme
- Vitamin B6 (pyridoxine)
- Zinc, magnesium and calcium supplements
- Evening primrose oil
- Yoga
- Homeopathy
- Hypnosis
- Acupuncture
- Reflexology
- Aromatherapy
- Lifestyle changes
- Analgesics
- Royal jelly
- Multivitamins
- Vitamin E

Research by Golub (1992) found that women who experienced severe psychological symptoms had lower self-esteem, experienced more stress in their lives, displayed more angry feelings and had less effective coping skills. This clearly has implications for the psychological treatment of women who seek therapy for PMS. Women with mild-to-moderate symptoms may benefit from simple advice about dietary changes and the lifestyle recommendations listed in Box 6.10. Basic advice should include encouragement to reduce external stress during the pre-menstrual phase, whilst regular exercise can help to reduce stress and tension. An added advantage of a dietary and lifestyle approach is that it gives the woman something positive to do and helps her to gain some control over her problems.

Box 6.10: Dietary and lifestyle recommendations (Mascarenas, 1990; Stewart et al., 1992; Hickerton, 1994)

- Reduce the intake of sugar and junk foods as high levels increase body fluids. Eat small portions every 3 hours to alleviate PMS symptoms
- Reduce salt intake as high levels increase body fluids
- Reduce the intake of caffeine, which contributes to anxiety and insomnia
- Limit the intake of animal fats. These produce a fall in circulating oestrogen and lactogenic hormones
- Advise good-quality vegetable oil, margarine and sunflower oil
- Encourage a diet high in vitamin-rich foods, such as vegetables, salad, fruit, liver, milk and eggs daily
- Limit the use of tobacco and alcohol as their harmful effects include a decrease in the balance of many vitamins and minerals
- Take regular exercise to reduce stress and increase feelings of well-being.
- Supplements advised are:
  - B6, E and multivitamins;
  - magnesium and calcium;
  - evening primrose oil

Various interventions that have shown positive results include supplementation with vitamin B6, which is reported to be mildly deficient in 15 per cent of the population (Stewart et al., 1992). B6 deficiency causes depression and fatigue, and has been associated with low progesterone levels (Mascerenas, 1990). Women should be encouraged to eat foods rich in vitamin B6, which include liver, eggs and milk).

Stewart et al. (1992) discussed research speculating that the relationship between oestrogen and B6 involves altered tissue distribution and perhaps enhances the body's need for vitamin B6. They also examined the effects of vitamin combinations. Combining B6 with magnesium and multivitamins has moderate efficacy, whilst vitamin B6 and zinc apparently influence other aspects of hormone metabolism in PMS sufferers. Vitamin E in high doses can be effective in reducing depression and anxiety, while evening primrose oil reduces breast symptoms.

If no significant improvement is shown after self-administration of the above measures, the woman must be advised to consult the general practitioner.

Nurses have a responsibility to provide information to help women to understand their PMS symptoms and offer behavioural strategies through support groups. This therapy helps some women to discover their own powers of self-determination. Although this task is not simple, it is certainly aided by the greater acceptance and understanding of the problems that women experience with this condition.

The nurse must serve as an advocate and initiate life management skills that would either supplement, or provide an alternative to, hormone and other drug therapies. To provide this service, the nurse must be knowledgeable in womens' health. The following measures are often helpful:

- sympathetic discussion of the problems and appropriate advice on the reorganization of aspects of life for those women who are feeling low;
- attention to general health, particularly nutrition, exercise, weight, sleep and relaxation.

Specific measures include:

- the control of fluids, salt and caffeine (Booth, 1995);
- herbal and vitamin remedies (Mascarenas, 1990);
- pyridoxine (vitamin B6) and gamma-linolenic acid (evening primrose oil), which can be helpful to some women (Henshaw and Smith, 1993);
- prescribed medication if none of the simpler measures is successful.

Perseverance on the part of both patient and nurse is necessary, and a number of different remedies and approaches may be used before a particular combination is found to be suitable. However, the dramatic improvement in the quality of life of the sufferer when a solution is found is worth the time and trouble taken in attempting to find a solution that alleviates pre-menstrual symptoms.

Summary

The treatment of PMS is most likely to be successful if the sufferer is shown care and understanding. There are a wide range of treatment approaches available. Women may initially benefit from exploring the role of social, nutritional and lifestyle factors, a strategy that may prove to be most effective and harmless. Most practice nurses are experienced in promoting healthy lifestyles, so PMS management would appear to be an extension of their current skills. It is, however, essential to recognize when initial home management is ineffective and to refer for consideration of other methods of treatment.

Failure to progress in controlling symptoms with any method of treatment after 2–3 months should prompt careful reassessment, which may include referral to a gynaecologist or psychiatrist.

The nurse must be a resource to inform women who have PMS symptoms and reassure them that PMS can be successfully treated through lifestyle changes, drug therapies or a combination of both.

Key points:

1. PMS is a recognized medical condition.
2. PMS must not be mistaken for a psychiatric disorder.
3. Women need empathetic support.
4. PMS symptoms can be reduced by lifestyle changes.

References

Andrews G (1994) Constructive advice for a poorly understood problem. Treatment and management of PMS. Professional Nurse 9(6): 364–79.

Bell JE, Dixon L, Sehy YS (1997) cited by Watson R, Mostly men. In Getliffe K and Dolman M (Eds) Promoting Continence in Clinical and Research Resource. London: Baillière Tindall pp 107–37.

Bernstein B, Kane R (1981) Physicians' attitudes towards female patients. Medical Care 19(6): 600.

Booth L (1995) Premenstrual syndrome: whose problem? Practice Nursing 6(20): 39–41.

Bradford J, Ryan C, Rothblum ED (1994) National lesbian health care survey: implications for mental health care. Journal of Consulting and Clinical Psychology 62(2): 228–42.

Brown P (1994) cited by Colbarn D, Assessment of the individual. In Colbarn D (Ed.) Promotion of Continence in Adult Nursing, 1st Edn, pp. 35–53. London: Chapman & Hall.

Cardozo L, Cutner A, Wise B (1993) Basic Urogynaecologoy. Oxford: Oxford University Press.

Cleave M (1991) The dark incontinence. Daily Telegraph 20 August: 13.

Colborn D (1994) The Promotion of Continence in Adult Nursing. London: Chapman & Hall.

Council on Scientific Affairs (1996) Health care needs of gay men and lesbians in the United States. Journal of the American Medical Association 275(17): 1354–9.

Creith E (1996) Undressing Lesbian Sex: Popular Images, Private Acts and Public Consequences. London: Cassell.

Dalton K (1980) Cyclical criminal acts in premenstrual syndrome. Lancet 2: 1070–1.

Department of Health (1977) Standards of Nursing Care – Promotion of Continence, of Management, of Incontinence. CNO SNC77/1. London: HMSO.

Donald I (1979) Practical Obstetric Problems. London: Lloyd-Luke.

Dorsey Green G (1987) Lesbian mothers: mental health considerations. In Bozett FW (Ed) Gay and Lesbian Parents. New York: Praeger Publishers.

Duffin H, Castleden C (1986) The continence nurse advisor's role in the British health care system. Clinics in Geriatric Medicine 2(4): 841.

Eliason M (1992) Cultural diversity in nursing care: the lesbian, gay, or bisexual client. Journal of Transcultural Nursing 5(1): 14–20.

Freud S (1920) Beyond the Pleasure Principle. London: Hogarth Press.

Glynn O (1993) Talk about menstrual problems. Practice Nurse 1(14): 889–92.

Golub S (1992) Periods from Menarche to Menopause. London: Sage.

Gould D (1990) Nursing Care of Women. London: Prentice Hall.

Haldeman DC (1994) The practice and ethics of sexual orientation conversion therapy. Journal of Consulting and Clinical Psychology 62(2): 221–7.

Hawton K, Oppenheimer C (1993) Sexual problems. In McPherson A (Ed.) Women's Problems in General Practice, 3rd Edn, p. 338. Oxford: Oxford University Press.

Henshaw C, Smith A (1993) The premenstrual syndrome: an occupational health issue. Occupational Health Review 45: 16–18.

Hickerton M (1994) Premenstrual syndrome. Practice Nursing 15(18): 18–20.

Hitchcock JM, Wilson HS (1992) Personal risking: lesbian self disclosure of sexual orientation to professional health care providers. Nursing Research 41(3): 178–83.

Hopkins J (1969) The lesbian personality. British Journal of Psychiatry 115: 1433–6.

Kliejnen J, Ter Iriet G, Knipschild P (1990) Vitamin B6 in the treatment of premenstrual syndrome: a review. British Journal of Obstetrics and Gynaecology 97: 847–52.

LesBeWell (1994) Findings of Research into Lesbian Health in Birmingham. Unpublished document.

Mandelstam D (1989) Understanding Incontinence. London: Chapman & Hall.

Mascarenas K (1990) What is premenstrual syndrome? Help and support for women with premenstrual syndrome. Professional Nurse 6(2): 72–5.

Mathiason A (1992) A clinical news. Nursing Standard 6(23): 15.

Millard J (1992) Continence in Primary Care. Australia: Continence Foundation of Australia.

Moos RH (1968) The development of a menstrual distress questionnaire. Psychosomatic Medicine 30: 853–67.

Newton C (1991) In Roper N, Logan W, Tierney A (Eds) Model in Action. London: Macmillan.

Norton C (1988) Continence can be presented at all ages. Professional Nurse 4(1): 22–6.

O'Brien PM (1987) Premenstrual Syndrome. London: Blackwell Scientific Publications.

O'Brien PM (1993) Helping women with premenstrual syndrome. British Medical Journal 307: 1471–5.

Rankow EJ (1995) Lesbian health issues for the primary health care provider. Journal of Family Practice 40(5): 486–92.

Sampson GA (1984) The role of the psychiatrist in the treatment of premenstrual syndrome. Maternal and Child Health 9(3): 96–101.

Savin Williams R (1994) Verbal and physical abuse as stressors in the lives of lesbian, gay male and bisexual youths. Journal of Consulting and Clinical Psychology 62(2): 261–9.

Scrambler A, Scrambler C (1985) Menstrual symptoms. Attitudes and consulting behaviour. Journal of Social Science and Medicine 20(1): 1065–8.

SHADY (1996) The Sexual Health of Women who Have Sex with Women in Merseyside and Cheshire. Specialist Health Promotion Service for South and East Cheshire. (unpublished)..

Siegelman M (1972) Adjustment of homosexual and heterosexual women. British Journal of Psychiatry 120: 477–81.

Simkin R (1991) Lesbians face unique health care problems. Canadian Medical Association Journal 145(12): 1620–3.

Smith & Nephew (1992) Continence in Primary Care. A Resource Pack. London: Continence Foundation.

Stevens PE (1992) Lesbian health care research: a review of the literature from 1970–1990. In Stern N (Ed.) Lesbian Health: What Are the Issues? San Francisco: Taylor & Francis: 1–27.

Stewart AC, Stewart M, Tooley S (1992) Premenstrual syndrome: is there a basis for a holistic approach? Maternal and Child Health 17(3): 86–8.

Sutherland FN (1990) Psychological aspects of premenstrual tension. Maternal and Child Health 15(12): 362–3.

Taylor RW (1983) Premenstrual syndrome. Proceedings of a workshop held at the Royal College of Obstetricians and Gynaecologists. London: Medical News Tribute.

Thomas T, Plymat K, Blannin J, Meade T (1980) Prevalence of urinary incontinence. British Medical Journal 281: 1243–5.

Woods NF, Taylor D, Mitchell ES, Lentz MJ (1992) Premenstrual symptoms and health seeking behaviour. Western Journal of Nursing Research 14(4): 418–43.

Further information

Dykenosis, a national bimonthly lesbian health news magazine. Available from PO Box 4048, King's Heath, Birmingham B14 7EF.

Lesbian Health Matters – Training Video. Available from London Lesbians in Health Care, The Wheel, Wild Court, off Kingsway, London WC2B 4AU.

Wilton T (1997) Good for You: A Handbook on Lesbian Health and Wellbeing. London: Cassell.

Useful addresses

Association of Continence Advice
The Basement,
2 Doughty Street,
London WC1N 2PH

Continence Foundation
380–384 Harrow Road,
London W9 2HU

Enuresis Resource and Information Centre (ERIC)
65 St Michael's Hill,
Bristol BS2 8D2

Disablement Income Group (DIG)
Millmead Business Centre,
Millard Road,
London N17 9QU

Disabled Living Centre
260 Broad Street,
Birmingham B1 2HF

Disabled Living Foundation Association of Continence Advisers
Disabled Living Foundation,
380–384 Harrow Road,
London W9 2HU

International Incontinence Society
c/o Mr Paul Abrams,
Department of Urology,
Southmead Hospital,
Bristol BS10 5NB

National Action on Incontinence
4 St Pancras Way,
London NW1 OPE

Sexual and Personal Relationships of the Disabled (SPOD)
286 Camden Road,
London N7 0BJ

Chapter 7
Health needs of young people

Wendy Cieslik, Susan Jones and Carol Atton

Young people receive most of their health education through school and/or from their parents. They do, however, present in the surgery for support and advice on a variety of health issues, particularly diet and sexual health.

Young people will continue to have sex, with or without health care support. Practice nurses must appreciate the implications of sexual activity for young people, so that they can offer an environment that welcomes young people and respects their maturity in seeking advice.

A parent may bring a child for dietary advice, expecting the nurse to achieve miracles in altering the child's dietary lifestyle. Many of the parents' expectations are, however, unrealistic. The second section of this chapter includes nutritional issues that are related to healthy eating within young people's lifestyles.

The nurse has an important role in identifying eating disorders, for which guidance on management and referral is offered in the final part of the chapter.

Young people appear to think that they are immune to the effects of poor diet and an unhealthy lifestyle. Health professionals must use any opportunity to encourage this client group to respect their bodies and reduce their morbidity.

Teenage health care

Many young people have no interest in their health, which makes the health professional's role extremely challenging. To them, ill-health occurs in old age, i.e. in their parents and those over 40! Promoting healthy lifestyles for young people will reduce morbidity and premature mortality, although the effects of health education cannot always be assessed in the short term.

One teenage male patient said, 'Well, I don't want to get old anyway, so I'll enjoy myself now.' As parents, many readers will relate to this comment and appreciate the difficulties of approaching teenage health issues.

Health promotion will often be opportunistic when the young person presents with an acute problem or for routine immunization or travel advice, and will supplement advice already given in school or at home. Parents appear less enthusiastic to discuss sexual health with their children, perhaps because they hope that the need will not arise. Practice nurses can fill this void through informed and sensitive advice and support. The following text emphasizes the rationale for young people's health needs to be included in any health agenda but leaves it to the reader to plan the approach best suited to each locality.

Young person's clinic

Specific clinics for teenagers are difficult to establish, but some young people do respond to the interest of health workers, particularly if they have a specific problem that needs addressing.

Local needs must be identified before attempting to establish a young person's clinic within general practice (see Chapter 4). Provision and energies can then be directed appropriately. Clinics can be run two ways: either by invitation or as a 'drop-in' service. A drop-in facility enables any emergency (for example, emergency contraceptive needs) to be dealt with immediately.

The many issues that the nurse and/or young person may wish to discuss are listed in Box 7.1. General lifestyle advice relating to smoking, alcohol, diet and exercise is pertinent to everyone, regardless of age, and should be tailored to the individual. It would also be naive to exclude recreational drugs and sexual health from the agenda.

Health professionals must be alert to girls who exercise excessively and/or have a low dietary calcium level, both of which are recognized risk factors for the development of osteoporosis. Eating disorders are discussed in detail later in the chapter.

It is essential that the nurse can make the young person feel comfortable and gain his or her confidence. The nurse who lives in the locality can find this both an advantage and a disadvantage, especially if she has teenage children. The young person may be embarrassed discussing issues with the parent of a friend: he or she has to be sure that the nurse will maintain confidentiality.

Box 7.1: Health issues for young people

- Current health status
- Smoking status
- Alcohol consumption
- Recreational drugs
- Exercise: amount and type
- Dietary advice: weight control, vegetarianism and calcium intake
- Family history: hyperlipidaemia, coronary heart disease, breast and cervical cancer, and testicular cancer
- Breast awareness and self-examination (girls)
- Testicular cancer and self-examination (boys)
- Acne
- Relationship problems
- Bullying
- School pressures
- Sexual health: contraception and emergency contraception, sexually transmitted diseases and safer sex
- Any 'taboo' topics the person may not wish to discuss with family or peers

---

Research has shown that boys in particular have low levels of knowledge about contraception, reproduction and contraceptive services (Winn et al., 1995). This highlights the importance of education for both boys and girls.

Many areas of health promotion are included within the National Curriculum and should be discussed throughout a child's school years. This may involve a multidisciplinary approach by school nurses, health visitors and/or family planning nurses. The level of interest and input will vary between and within regions and schools.

Practice nurses may have little influence over most general lifestyle changes but may influence the sexual health of young people by offering a sensitive, confidential health clinic. A small-scale survey carried within the author's practice and locality highlighted the poor uptake of contraceptive services (Box 7.2).

Ideally, the practice would supply a teenager-friendly waiting room specifically for young people, with posters and leaflets applicable to youth, although realistically few practices could find the space to meet this ideal. Posters on safe sex and condom use may offend some older patients, as well as some staff, and are seldom seen in general waiting areas.

The responses of a random sample of high-school pupils suggest that teenagers are interested in a health clinic if timed during the weekend (Box 7.2). Practices that wish to develop this service will have to be flexible and accommodating to clients' demands.

Box 7.2: Results of a local survey (Cieslik, 1995, unpublished data)

The request for contraceptive advice/methods within one general practice and family planning clinic were examined. The locality is semi-rural and comprises primarily social groups II–IIIM

Within the surgery (practice population 7600):

- under 16s – 3 were on combined oral contraception and 4 had requested emergency contraception

Within the local family planning clinic:

- under 16s – 1 visited and none requested emergency contraception

A small survey of 20 local high school pupils was carried out to determine interest in the establishment of a teenage health clinic:

- not interested – 6;
- interested – 14, of whom 9 stated that Saturday was their preferred day

Pupils felt that they could approach their 'in-house' nurse for any advice they needed

---

Teenage sexual health clinic

General practices should offer a non-judgemental sexual health service for those young people who require advice and support. The many consequences of early sexual activity are listed in Box 7.3.

Sex education is a vital element in the care of both the sexually active teenager and the teenager contemplating sexual activity. A teenage sexual health clinic should have clear aims, which may include:

- providing a user-friendly environment;
- providing user-friendly terminology;

Box 7.3: Consequences of early sexual activity

- Sexually transmitted diseases, including HIV, hepatitis B and genital herpes
- Unplanned pregnancy, with associated emotional and physical trauma (see Chapter 4)
- Cervical neoplasia
- Exploitation
- Psychological trauma

- giving holistic advice regarding aspects of general health care;
- encouraging responsibility in sexual matters;
- stressing that confidentiality will be maintained (see Chapter 1).

Sexual health is an important issue at any age, but the teenage years are of special importance in ensuring a healthy and well-informed adult population. This was identified by the Conservative government and included as a Health of the Nation target that aimed to reduce the rate of conception amongst the under 16s by at least 50 per cent by the year 2000 – from 9.5 per 1000 girls aged 13–15 years in 1989 to no more than 4.8 per 1000 girls (DoH, 1992).

Although this target has been excluded from the Labour party's recent Green Paper 'Our Healthier Nation' (DoH, 1998), health workers must continue their efforts to reduce the number of conceptions in schoolgirls.

> **Activity 7.1: Compare the number of under-16 pregnancies within your practice during a stated time (e.g. during 1998) with that of another district and nationally. Consider the implications of your findings.**

Teenage pregnancy

The UK has the highest teenage pregnancy rate in Western Europe. Since 1990, the pregnancy rate in 16–19-year-olds decreased to a rate of 56.8 per 1000 in 1997 (NHS Centre for Reviews and Dissemination, 1997). The under-16 pregnancy rate has remained constant over the past 20 years at 8.3 per 1000 (Office of National Statistics, 1996). In 1993, district variations in teenage pregnancy rate ranged from 4.2 to 19.3 per 1000 (OPCS, 1993).

Risk factors associated with teenage pregnancy

Several important issues associated with teenage pregnancy were highlighted in a recent report (NHS Centre for Reviews and Dissemination, 1997). Teenagers who live in deprived areas with fewer welfare services have higher pregnancy rates, and the proportion of pregnancies terminated is lower than that in more affluent areas. This may explain the wide variation in teenage pregnancy rates between districts. Those who continue with their pregnancy, particularly those under 16, and keep their children have been shown to be at higher risk of adverse educational, social and health outcomes.

Daughters of mothers who had a teenage pregnancy appear more likely to become teenage mothers themselves (Seamark and Gray, 1997). A small controlled study supporting this theory involved 31 girls who had had at least one teenage pregnancy. The mother's pregnancy history was also established. The planned pregnancies were not terminated (Table 7.1).

Table 7.1: A study into teenage pregnancy (Seamark and Gray, 1997)

	Mother had teenage pregnancy	Number Planned	Pregnancy continued	Pregnancy terminated
Yes	16	5	5	6
No	15	1	2	12

Ashken and Soddy (1980) and Wilson (1980) noted other elements of deprivation and teenage pregnancy (Box 7.4).

Box 7.4: Elements associated with deprivation and teenage pregnancy

- Teenagers living in care, or having left care, have higher teenage pregnancy rates than those who live at home
- School non-attendees (girls who are excluded or who truant)
- Homeless or runaway teenagers
- Poor awareness of, and access to, contraceptive services, health services and sex education
- Individual characteristics, i.e. low self-esteem, first intercourse, maturity and knowledge
- Poor educational achievement

Adverse outcomes associated with teenage pregnancy

Ranjan (1993) reported that teenage girls are at risk of higher morbidity and mortality during pregnancy. The extremes of reproductive life are most harmful in relation to maternal, fetal and neonatal risk. Conception under the age of 16 is associated with an increased perinatal death rate, over 18 per cent of premature deliveries occurring in this group. The effects on both mother and child are examined separately, although some issues are relevant to both.

The young mother

Teenage conception can adversely affect the mother-to-be in several ways, including education and economic status.

The health of the young teenage mother is compromised by obstetric complications, including hypertension, anaemia, placental abruption and depression. Termination of pregnancy has its own associated physical and psychological problems.

It is common for the girl to drop out of school when pregnant. Even if the girl returns to school, there will be gaps in her education, which will ultimately affect her long-term employment prospects.

Socio-economic effects include reduced employment opportunities, decreased independence and increased dependence on the welfare state. Housing and nutrition are likely to be poor.

The child

The child of a teenage mother has an increased risk of hospitalization as a result of non-accidental injury, sudden infant death syndrome, prematurity, experiencing abuse and becoming a pregnant teenager. The child is also at risk of preschool developmental delays and, as poverty is more prevalent, may suffer from poor nutrition and poor housing.

A review of research into adverse outcomes is summarized by the NHS Centre for Reviews and Dissemination (1997).

There will always be exceptions to the examples given above, and some young mothers will have healthy pregnancies and be well supported by their families.

Prevention of teenage pregnancy

Educational approach

Despite the diverse approaches that have been used in the delivery of sex education, a number of distinct characteristics have emerged. Many studies have demonstrated consistent evidence that sex and contraceptive education within school settings does not increase sexual activity or rates of pregnancy (Frost and Forrest, 1995; Peersman et al., 1996). In fact, the opposite is highlighted. A service providing accurate information about sex and contraception, knowing when and how to access contraceptive services, appears to be the essential ingredient in the success of educational programmes. Four school-based educational models for the delivery of approaches to preventing teenage pregnancy have been evaluated (NHS Centre for Reviews and Dissemination, 1997):

- *Abstinence programmes*: The main aim is delayed sexual activity until later in the teenage years or until marriage. This was found not to have any effect on delaying sexual activity or reducing pregnancy rates.
- *Skills building combined with factual information*: Postponement of sexual activity is stressed, combined with factual information on contraceptives and how to access contraception services. This approach was found to have some success in terms of changes in both sexual activity and contraceptive behaviour.
- *School-based programmes that are linked to contraceptive services*: Sex education along with access to contraceptive services proved successful in increasing the use of contraceptives.
- *School-based and school-linked clinics*: Studies in the USA have shown inconsistent results.

In the UK, the Department of Health (DoH) leaves primary responsibility for sexual and emotional education to parents. Any teaching offered by schools should be complementary to or 'supportive' of that of parents and show 'regard to parents' views' regarding content and presentation. The implementation of Section 241 of the Education Act 1993 (DfE, 1994) allows parents to remove their children from all parts of a school's sex education programme. Young people may therefore be withdrawn from sex education sessions irrespective of their own wishes. This contradicts aspects of the Children's Act (1989), for example autonomy.

Within general practice, facilities exist for young people to access confidential help and advice regarding all aspects of sexual health, contraception and emergency contraception, the most accessible and appropriate person being the family planning-trained practice nurse.

Research has highlighted that, regardless of from whom or from where young people get their sex education, a very important aspect to consider is *when* it is given. It has been demonstrated that changing sexual and contraceptive behaviour is less successful when young people have already commenced sexual activity before the programme starts (NHS Centre for Reviews and Dissemination, 1997).

Winfield (1995) suggests several reasons why teenagers deserve special attention from family planning services:

- the lack of sex education for primary school children, making a rescue package at puberty essential;

- mixed messages from the media and adult population: romance and sex are offered as the ultimate for self-fulfilment, but teenagers are denied access to contraceptive advice and criticized if they are sexually active;
- teenagers fear criticism and are ignorant of the law, which can exclude them from sources of help.

A Family Planning Factsheet (Family Planning Association, 1994) detailed a small-scale survey of 1000 young people aged 16 and under, who were asked what they needed from a family planning service. Five main areas were noted (Box 7.5).

Box 7.5: What young people need from a family planning service (Family Planning Association, 1994)

- Family planning services should be easy to get to (93.1%)
- Staff should be friendly (91.7%)
- No appointment should be needed (86%)
- A telephone helpline should be available (83.2%)
- Friends should be able to come along too (80%)

Allen (1991), reporting on Policy Studies Institute findings, stated that over 90 per cent of the teenagers interviewed were worried about visiting their general practitioner for contraception. They saw general practitioners as gruff, abrupt and disapproving, with little time to discuss their problems and the range of contraceptive options other than the pill that was available, or to explain how to use a contraceptive method correctly. The main concern, however, was that the consultation would not be confidential.

Emergency contraception

Emergency contraception, also known as post-coital contraception, is an extremely effective and safe method of avoiding pregnancy following unprotected intercourse or method failure, or a default or method accident in pill-taking.

The two methods available are hormonal (emergency contraceptive pills) and the intrauterine device (IUD). The former is the most common method used for the young person. Insertion of an IUD may prove difficult in a woman who has not been pregnant and is unsuitable for those at high risk of sexually transmitted disease. However, the risk of unintended pregnancy should be weighed against these risks, notably because the IUD is so effective.

Confidentiality

The duty of confidentiality to any person under the age of 16 is as great as that for any adult. The legal position relating to contraception to under 16s was verified in the House of Lord's ruling in the Gillick case (1985). This established that people aged under 16 who are able fully to understand the proposed treatment and its implications are competent to consent to medical treatment regardless of age. The doctor is, however, legally obliged to discuss the value of parental involvement and encourage the young person to inform a parent. If the girl declines, she must be assured that her confidentiality will be respected.

The doctor must assess whether the young person understands the potential risks and benefits of treatment, whether intercourse is likely with or without contraception and whether physical or mental health is likely to suffer without contraceptive provision or advice. The doctor must also be sure that it is in the young person's best interest to provide contraception.

Young people who are made aware of these issues may be more confident to approach health professionals for contraceptive advice. This is perhaps the fundamental hurdle that must be overcome before a substantial reduction in teenage pregnancy will be seen.

> **Activity 7.2: Discuss with colleagues how contraceptive services within your practice could be more 'user friendly' to encourage young people to access them.**

Special issues relating to young people

Many teenage pregnancies could be avoided if girls were more aware of emergency contraception, including where to obtain it, how to use it and the issues of confidentiality.

The young person should be treated with the same respect as a member of any other client group. She will probably require more support than adults as she may experience feelings of shame, fear, embarrassment or guilt. All or any of these emotions will need to be identified and managed in a positive and sympathetic manner. The young person who can feel confident and relaxed once the consultation has begun will, it is hoped, feel less negative about her situation and realize that she has made a mature decision in seeking advice. This will enable her to deal with her situation in a more positive manner.

The nurse who has a trusting rapport with a girl is more likely to establish a basis for future consultations, which will allow future problems to be discussed more freely. The approachability of the nurse will be disseminated amongst her peers; hence a successful first consultation is paramount.

There have been no reported deaths resulting from the use of emergency contraceptive methods (oral communication, FPA, January 1998). Emergency contraceptive pills have no age-related contraindications.

Research suggests that many young people have an inadequate knowledge of the method of use of emergency contraception (Graham et al., 1996). The term 'morning after pill' is commonly used, but this causes confusion as it suggests that the treatment required must be immediate rather than the 72 hours for the oral route and five days for IUD insertion; thus clear, concise advice must be given. Even when the young woman has knowledge, she may find it difficult to obtain emergency contraception for several reasons (Box 7.6). Some girls may need services within school hours, particularly if they are dependent on school transport. Others will prefer after-school services. General practices can provide contraceptive services to girls who are registered elsewhere. This knowledge may increase the uptake of contraceptive services as confidentiality is often a girl's major concern.

Box 7.6: Barriers to young people accessing services (Graham et al., 1996)

The young person:

- may not know where to find family planning services;
- may not have the confidence to insist on an emergency appointment;
- may be unaware of confidentiality.

Clinic times may not be outside school hours, so access will be difficult

---

Young men

It would appear from the above text that sexual health advice and contraception are the domain of girls, but young men also have a responsibility to prevent pregnancy. This should be considered for all health promotion initiatives. It may be appropriate to encourage boys to attend family planning or sexual health clinics. This would offer an opportunity to discuss sexually transmitted disease, contraception and emergency contraception.

Sexual health advice should not be aimed solely at heterosexual couples. Young men who have sex with men also require sexual health advice (see Chapter 5).

Young men often lead lifestyles that make their parents despair. Advice on healthy eating, smoking, alcohol consumption, recreational drugs and general health is often ignored. Health professionals must try to tailor their advice to suit the lifestyes of modern youth, in an effort to reduce the damage to health.

Summary

The need for a facility for young people within general practice has been highlighted within this text. In order for this facility to be successful, it needs to incorporate all the issues previously discussed. Teenage health clinics also offer an opportunity to discuss the management of chronic conditions such as epilepsy, asthma and hayfever.

The young person must be treated with respect and be offered sound, accurate information. Accessibility of services must be ensured, and the assurance of confidentiality can help in establishing the success of the service. Where a rapport exists between nurse and young person, opportunities will arise for further health promotion.

Key points:

1. Young people have health needs that must be recognized.
2. Teenage pregnancy has adverse social, educational and economic outcomes.
3. Confidentiality must be respected.
4. The sexual health of young men must be included in a health agenda.

Nutritional issues in young people

Adolescence is a time of both rapid physical growth and hormonal change. On average, a girl's growth spurt occurs between the ages of 10 and 13 and a boy's between 12 and 15. With increasing independence and money of their own, missed meals, snacking, cigarette smoking and alcohol consumption often become habits in teenage years. Peer pressure and self-identity are well known to be powerful influences on young people.

What is a healthy diet for a young person?

The current dietary recommendations for all age groups are based on dietary reference values (DRVs) (DoH, 1991). The range is divided into three different groups (Figure 7.1).

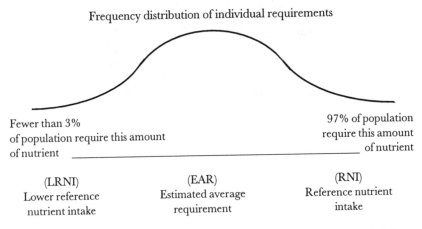

Frequency distribution of individual requirements

Fewer than 3%
of population require this amount
of nutrient

97% of population
require this amount
of nutrient

(LRNI)	(EAR)	(RNI)
Lower reference nutrient intake	Estimated average requirement	Reference nutrient intake

RNI is the figure commonly used, and is equivalent to the recommended daily allowance (RDA), which is still used on food labelling.

EAR is used for the daily energy requirement of a person, for example:

EAR	11–14 years	15–18 years
Girls	1845 kcal	2110 kcal
Boys	2200 kcal	2775 kcal

Figure 7.1: Dietary recommendations.

The remit of the Committee on the Medical Aspects of Food Policy (COMA) reports (DoH, 1989a, 1994) is to reduce the amount of heart disease and obesity through promoting diets containing less fat (to account for 35 per cent of total energy) and more carbohydrate (to make up 50 per cent of the total energy). The National Food Guide (Balance of Good Health) shown in Figure 7.2, also commonly known as the 'plate model', is the nationally recognized system used for teaching healthy eating recommendations. It was launched in 1994 after in-depth, qualitative research and development, including widespread consultation. The model's focus of food on a plate is flexible and aims to give the public a consistent, clear message on healthy eating based on research.

The actual amounts of food required vary greatly according to the individual and are indicated in the measures shown in Table 7.2 (p. 233). A detailed analysis of individual nutritional requirements can be

Fruit and vegetables   Bread, other cereals and potatoes

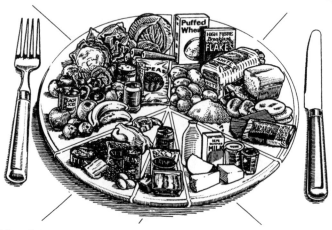

Meat, fish and alternatives   Foods containing fat   Milk and dairy foods
                                Foods containing sugar

Figure 7.2: The balance of good health (reproduced with kind permission of the Health Education Authority).

obtained from a state-registered dietitian. 'Helping People Change' courses run by health promotion units provide further training and information. Composite foods such as pizza, lasagne, pies and sandwiches fit into several of the groups: pizza, for example, fits into all five groups. The proportion of the food groups eaten daily is the key to making healthy choices.

What are young people eating? – food habits and nutrients at risk

Young people eat a lot more snacks than adults do (Johnson and Hackett 1997). The nutritional status of young people, based on their height and weight, is not a cause for concern, although children from low-income families are shorter than their more affluent peers (DoH, 1989b). However, in terms of preventing heart disease and other diseases, the present diet of many young people is unsatisfactory, comprising too much fat and insufficient micronutrients, i.e. the minerals, iron, calcium, zinc and copper, and the vitamins thiamin, riboflavin and B6.

The results of a comprehensive survey of teenage eating patterns will be published by the DoH and Ministry of Agriculture, Fisheries and Food (MAFF) in 1999. The most recent large-scale dietary survey of teenage eating habits is 'The Diets of British School Children' (DoH, 1989b). Its findings have been duplicated by several smaller surveys (HEA, 1995). The nutritionally at risk young people are summarized in Table 7.3 (page 234).

Table 7.2: What is a measure?

Food groups	Suggested daily amounts and types of food
Bread and cereals	6–14 measures One measure = 1 slice bread, 2 heaped tablespoons boiled rice or pasta, 1 small chapatti or 2 egg-sized potatoes
Fruit and vegetables	5 or more portions a day 1 portion = 1 piece fresh fruit (i.e. apple or orange) or 1 medium portion of vegetables, including salad Fresh/tinned/frozen/dried fruit and vegetables are all included to dispel the myth that these are inferior to fresh ones
Meat fish and alternatives	2–4 measures One measure = 3 medium slices of meat or fish, 4 tablespoons of lentils or dhal Choose low-fat meats and low-fat cooking methods Choose oily fish, e.g. mackerel or salmon, once a week
Milk and dairy products	3–5 measures* One measure = 1 medium glass milk or 1 pot of yoghurt
Foods containing fat	1–5 measures One measure = 1 teaspoon of butter, margarine or oil, 1 packet of crisps or 1 tablespoon of mayonnaise
Foods containing sugar	0–2 measures One measure = 2 biscuits, 1 small bar of chocolate, 1 small bag of sweets, half a slice of cake or 3 teaspoons of sugar

*Increased for young people as calcium requirements during adolescence are higher. Reproduced with permission from HEA (1997).

Teenage pregnancy

Teenage pregnancy increases nutritional demands, especially if the mother herself is still growing. The major nutrients at risk are calcium, iron, zinc and folic acid. These are provided by all the food groups except fatty and sugary foods. Food safety also requires careful consideration during pregnancy. Further information can be obtained from the local Environmental Health Department.

Calcium

The reference nutrient intake (RNI) for calcium is 1000 mg daily for 11–18-year-old boys and 800 mg for girls of the same age. This is achieved by eating a combination of the exchanges listed in Table 7.4 (page 235).

Table 7.3: Nutritionally at risk young people aged 11–16 years

At-risk group	Nutrients at risk	Food groups to provide adequate nutrients
All	Protective levels of micronutrients, especially those in fruit and vegetables*	Fruit and vegetables: five portions per day
All	Too much fat	More fruit and vegetables More bread and cereals in place of fatty foods
All girls over 14 years old	Calcium	Milk and dairy products Bread and cereals
Girls who are dieting, Some vegetarians who do not choose a suitable meat substitute	Iron	Meat, fish and alternatives- Bread and cereals Sources of vitamin C, e.g. fruit and vegetables
Young people from low-income families	Riboflavin	Milk and dairy products Bread and cereals Green leafy vegetables
Young people from ethnic groups	Micronutrients Energy	Meat, fish and alternatives Bread and cereals Fruit and vegetables Wide variety of all groups, particularly bread and cereals

*Twenty-five per cent had eaten no fruit and 33% no vegetables on the previous day (Hackett et al., 1997)

Milk and milk products have a much higher concentration of calcium than all other foods, and the calcium is more readily absorbed than from other sources. About 45 per cent of adult skeletal mass is formed during adolescence. A low calcium intake of less than 500 mg calcium a day may reduce bone peak bone mass and increase the risk of osteoporosis (National Dairy Council, 1992).

As 60 per cent of 14-year-old girls have an intake less than the RNI of calcium, girls must be strongly encouraged to eat more calcium in order to protect their bones. Non-milk drinking young people need to be advised to eat extra sources of calcium, for example fortified soya milk, white bread and cheese. Load-bearing exercise, such as walking, aids bone formation and is yet another good reason for promoting regular physical activity.

Table 7.4: 200 mg calcium exchanges (McCance and Widdowson, 1991)

Food	Portion
Milk – all types	180 ml/6 fl oz
Yoghurt – all types	120 g/4 oz average pot
Hard cheese, e.g. cheddar	30 g/1 oz
Cottage cheese – lower in calcium	270 g/10 oz
Fromage frais	240 g/8 oz
White bread (calcium content of wholemeal bread varies; refer to label)	200 g/7 oz, i.e. 6 slices
Canned salmon if eat the bones	240 g/8 oz, i.e. 5 average salmon sandwiches
Cooked broccoli	500 g/20 oz, i.e. 4 large portions

Iron

The daily RNI for iron for 11–18-year-old boys is 11.3 mg and that for girls of the same age 14.8 mg. This is achieved by a combination of the iron exchanges in Table 7.5.

Iron absorption is increased by the presence of haem iron, i.e. meats, and by vitamin C. It is decreased by the presence of tea, coffee and the phytates in fibre. The most highly absorbed sources of iron are red meat and liver. Nelson et al. (1993) found that 10 per cent of 12–14-year-old girls were anaemic, this being associated with a low intake of iron and vitamin C. As yet, it is unclear whether mild anaemia causes poorer physical health, behaviour and academic performance. There is strong evidence that anaemia during pregnancy results in hypertension and heart disease in adulthood (Godfrey et al., 1991).

The main sources of iron in the 12–14-year age group (Moynihan et al., 1994) are:

- Meat 19 per cent
- Breakfast cereals 15 per cent
- Bread 12 per cent
- Potatoes, including crisps and chips 11 per cent
- Drinks 7 per cent
- Bakery goods 7 per cent

Table 7.5: Iron exchanges of 2.5 mg iron (McCance and Widdowson, 1991, 1996)

Food	Portion
Roast red meat, i.e. beef, lamb and pork	100 g/3.5 oz – average portion
Beefburger	100 g/3.5 oz – 2½ average burgers
Corned beef	100 g/3.5 oz
Cooked liver	20 g/0.75 oz
Shepherds pie	360 g/13 oz – average portion
Egg	130 g/4.5 oz, i.e. 2 eggs
Tuna fish canned in oil	150 g/5.25 oz – large portion
Sardines canned in tomato sauce	85 g/3 oz – 3½ average sardines
Baked beans	200 g/7 oz – large portion
Dhal – cooked	90 g/3 oz – 2–3 tablespoons
Bran Flakes or Special K	20 g/0.75 oz – small portion
Average fortified breakfast cereal	40 g/1.5 oz – medium to large portion
White bread	150 g/5.5 oz – 4 medium slices
Wholemeal bread	90 g/3 oz – 2½ slices
Chappati	120 g/4.25 oz – 2 average

Overweight

The prevalence of overweight amongst the British population has risen dramatically in the past decade as our lifestyle has become more sedentary. This is becoming a major public health problem. The DOH (1995a) has stated that 48 per cent of adult women and 57 per cent of adult men are overweight (defined as a body mass index, BMI, above 25), a proportion that is rising out of control. Overweight children are twice as likely to become overweight adults, and there is a strong genetic influence in determining fatness. Physical activity can help to prevent obesity (Ottley, 1997).

BMI (weight/height^2) values in general practices are for people over 16 years old; BMI charts from birth to 23 years of age are available from the Child Growth Foundation. The accepted definition of overweight in young people is two or more major centiles above the height centile using the child growth charts. Overweight children are likely to be bullied at school, which compounds the problem.

The causes of overweight are a combination of insufficient habitual physical activity, an excess energy intake, especially from fat, and genetic, social and cultural factors. Fat calories are more fattening than carbohydrate calories. Levels of physical activity in young people have been shown to be nationally low, and females exercise less than males. Children from disadvantaged socio-economic backgrounds and Asian children, especially girls, do less exercise than other children (HEA, 1992).

The main aim of dietary advice in this age group is to establish regular eating patterns high in carbohydrates and to achieve static weight gain so that the young person grows into his or her weight. Once growth has stopped, the emphasis is still on establishing regular eating habits, with a maximum weight loss of 1–2 lb (0.5–1.0 kg) per week.

What can the practice nurse do?

- Use the plate model as a teaching tool and emphasize the choice of a wide variety from the main four food groups and a minimum of foods from the fatty and sugary group. This gets across the nutritional message that regular meals and the proportion of food on the plate are the key to losing weight. Strict dieting is inappropriate in this age group.
- Emphasize that diets high in carbohydrate achieve a lower fat diet, which helps to promote weight loss.
- Acknowledge that, to be successful, the young person needs to want to lose weight. He or she needs positive, continual support from family and friends.
- Discuss with the family their eating habits and ask them how these could be improved. Changes are more likely to be achieved if the young person and family suggest the changes. Three changes are a realistic aim.
- The widespread advertising and social acceptability of snack foods is a hindrance to long-term compliance to any weight-reducing diet. This needs to be acknowledged and discussed.
- Promote increased habitual physical activity – some leisure centres run exercise groups for overweight young people. Encourage walking.
- Discuss short-term goals with treats for achieving the agreed target weight and the alternative use of pocket money instead of snack foods.
- Liase with the local community dietitian, health promotion department and school nurses for further information; they may run a suitable slimming group.
- If the family agrees, consider referring to child psychologist when comfort eating or psychological problems are a big issue. Service provision varies between authorities.
- Offer regular follow-up as agreed with the client, with clear guidelines on discharge if goals are not being met.

The DoH (1989b) suggest that teenagers who are slimming may be deficient in essential vitamins and minerals, especially iron, which needs taking into account when discussing dieting with this age group.

Vitamins

There is no objective evidence that extra vitamins and minerals improve intelligence. A wide variety of foods from each food group ensures sufficient intake of vitamins and minerals (Nelson et al., 1990).

Vegetarianism

Vegetarianism has occurred throughout history for a variety of economic, religious, cultural and social reasons. The growing awareness of ecological issues may cause young people to stop eating animal foods. The Realeat survey (1997) found that 5 per cent of the adult population were vegetarians. The most recent Realeat survey of under-16s not eating meat was in 1988, when 9 per cent were vegetarian or avoided meat. Girls are more likely than boys to give up meat.

A well-planned vegetarian diet is a healthy way of eating, but without careful thought and planning, it is potentially inadequate during a period of rapid growth. It can easily become a focus of family discord, especially if meat is given up without considering an alternative. Vegetarian cooking often requires more planning and is an ideal opportunity for young people to develop their own cooking skills. There is an increasing variety of prepacked vegetarian meals available in supermarkets and health shops. Table 7.6 illustrates the nutrients that may be lacking in a vegetarian diet.

Suggestions for sandwich fillings

- Cheese and cucumber, or flavoured cheese spreads
- Nut butters, nut/lentil paté or hummous
- Yeast extract and tomato
- Egg
- Banana.

Suggestions for cooked meals

- *Meat substitutes*: Soya and Quorn can be used to make bolognese or chilli dishes served with rice or spaghetti and salad. Vegeburgers can be served with potato and various vegetables.

Table 7.6: The vegetarian way of eating – nutrients potentially at risk

Type of vegetarian	Nutrients that may be at risk
No meat	Iron, zinc
No meat or fish	Iron, zinc, omega-3 polyunsaturated fats in oily fish
Vegans: no meat, fish, eggs or milk	Iron, zinc, omega-3 polyunsaturated fats in oily fish, vitamin B12, calcium, riboflavin, possibly protein and energy if pulses and nuts are not used
Macrobiotic/fruitarian diet	All the above, protein and energy, trace elements; potentially a nutritional disaster

- *Beans*: Dishes made with beans (red, haricot, aduki, butter or baked beans), including mixed bean goulash and chilli.
- *Cheese*: Cauliflower cheese with pasta and vegetables; baked potato with cheese, baked beans and salad; cheese flan with vegetables/salad and baked potato.
- *Rice*: Bean paella, vegetable risotto, or rice served with lentil/dhal curry and chappatis.
- *Vegetable dishes*: Stir fry with noodles and pasta sauces (lasagne, spaghetti).

The key point is to have a balanced meal, with a mixture of food groups. It is also important to emphasize the importance of the following foods for:

- *iron*: fortified breakfast cereals, bread, chappatis and bulgar wheat; dark green vegetables such as broccoli, spinach and spring greens;
- *calcium*: calcium-fortified soya milks (usually sweetened) for vegan and macrobiotic/fruitarian diets; see above for a discussion of milk and dairy products;
- *zinc*: lentils, cheese and wholegrain cereals such as wholemeal breads and flours.

Vitamin B12 is found only in animal foods, including eggs and milk. It is absolutely essential that vegans and young people choosing to eat macrobiotic/fruitarian-type diets take a supplement or foods fortified with B12, for example Barmene, Tastex, fortified soya milk,

Protoveg or grapenuts. A frank deficiency of B12 and folate causes megaloblastic anaemia, which is highest amongst Asian vegetarians. Vitamin B12 deficiency has been reported in children fed Rastafarian macrobiotic diets and vegan diets. It is also advised that vegetarians may need to supplement their diet with vitamin B12, particularly during pregnancy and breastfeeding (Thomas, 1996).

> **Activity 7.3: How would you advise a mother who is worried about her 14-year-old daughter who has recently given up eating meat, fish and eggs?**

Food, health and low income

There are inequalities in health in the UK that are dependent on income (DoH, 1995b). This is reflected in the poorer quality of the diet in children from lower socio-economic groups, who eat less fruit and vegetables, drink less milk and eat more fatty and sugary foods than those from more affluent groups.

Poverty has grown rapidly in the 1980s. In 1979, one child in 10 lived in poverty, a figure that rose to one in four in 1990 (National Forum for Coronary Heart Disease Prevention, 1993). Poverty is defined by the EU as an income of less than half the average household earning – in today's money less than £115 week (Leather, 1996). Contrary to some publicity, healthy eating following the COMA recommendations costs more (Barratt, 1997). Surveys of the cost of healthy eating show that families on income support need to spend a higher proportion of their income on food to achieve the recommendations than does the rest of the population. Food costs more in poorer areas because shoppers are dependent on local shops rather than supermarkets.

Although local initiatives such as food co-operatives and 'Get Cooking' projects are addressing these issues, they are all insecurely funded. A lack of basic cooking and budgeting skills, particularly amongst people from disadvantaged economic backgrounds, is an area of great concern amongst health professionals (personal communication, local project, 1996). Government policies need to be altered so that the national curriculum includes everyday basic cooking and budgeting skills.

> **Activity 7.4: Make a directory of local contact points for food co-operatives and cooking projects. Consider the needs of your practice population (refer to Chapter 4).**

School meals

The provision of school meals has undergone several changes over the past 20 years. In 1980, the Education Act removed the obligation on local education authorities (LEAs) to provide school meals, except for children entitiled to free school meals (at the present time those families on income support). In 1988, the Local Government Act introduced complusory competitive tendering, and most secondary schools now have cash cafeteria systems (Passmore, 1997), although the standard of school meals has not improved. The school meals campaign and other organizations have been campaigning since 1992 to reintroduce national nutrition standards into school meals (Passmore, 1997). Nutritional standards for primary schools at the time of writing are at the Green Paper stage, with their implementation planned for 1999.

The Schools Nutrition Action Groups (SNAGs, 1994) and the 'Excellence in Schools' White Paper (DoE, 1997) have addressed the issue of whole school policies on food and nutrition, including the provision of healthy snack choices and breakfasts. This is the way forward in achieving healthier diets for young people as many schools currently offer high-fat and high-sugar snacks from vending machines and tuck shops to raise money for school funds.

Healthier alternatives could be provided that would also maximize financial return. SNAGs have achieved this in pilot studies:

> The key element is in building a school-based healthy alliance between pupils, staff and caterers so that decisions taken and solutions agreed are their own. (SNAGs, 1994)

Attitudes to food

It is well appreciated that the behaviour of friends and also self-identity influence young peoples' food and health choices. They do not take the long-term view that diet affects health. New codes of advertising practice and procedure could make healthy food choices easier; only 10 per cent of food advertisements aimed at children could currently be said to encourage a healthy diet (National Forum for Coronary Heart Disease Prevention, 1993). Also, as teenagers rely on snacks, the development of a greater choice of healthy snacks by the food industry would be a very positive influence on young people's diets.

To illustrate the huge financial divide between the aggressive marketing of many snack foods and that of fruit and vegetables, a recent campaign to market fruit and vegetables attracted financing of £0.5 million (Hackett et al., 1997); in contrast, the 1994 annual budget to market one brand of crisps (Walkers) was £6 million (company literature). The entire 1997–98 HEA budget for nutrition projects was £707, 000 in 1997.

Woodward et al. (1997) demonstrated that the more television young people watched, the less healthy their diet. The average daily television watching time was 3.3 hours. Thus, the time spent watching television seems to be a good indicator of poor diet if children watch over 3.3 hours daily.

Self-esteem-raising programmes have an important contribution in giving more vulnerable young people the skills to choose healthy foods and lifestyles. Some LEAs are organizing these courses.

Missing meals is common amongst young people: 20 per cent of 14–18-year-olds miss breakfast (National Dairy Council, 1989). However, regular breakfast eating is associated with lower fat intakes and increased micronutrients (Crawley, 1993). There is some evidence that missing breakfast adversely affects brain function in young people (Pollitt, 1995). Missing breakfast in nutritionally at-risk children has definite adverse effects on cognitive skills; in well-nourished children the effects are less clear.

Summary

The plate model provides a clear teaching tool to discuss food choices from a wide variety of food groups and the importance of the proportion of foods.

The young people most at risk of inadequate diets are those from low-income families, girls over 14 years old, some vegetarians, young people from ethnic groups, pregnant girls and those with low self-esteem. As snack foods play an important part in young people's nutrition, choosing healthy snacks and eating more fruit and vegetables are key nutritional messages that require changes in national policy. Liaison with community dietitians and the health promotion service will provide nurses with training and other resources.

In many instances, young people and their parents can be reassured that the diet is nutritionally sound, although unconventional by adult standards.

Eating disorders

Strange as it seems, eating disorders are not about food or weight but about feelings. Sufferers are deeply distressed. By concentrating all their energies on food and dieting, the eating disorder becomes a way of coping with emotional pain and turmoil. At first, dieting and weight loss provide a sense of achievement and control over one's life that gives relief from difficult feelings or intolerable dilemmas, but when the ill-effects of starvation, frequent bingeing and/or purging become apparent, the eating disorder itself becomes the dominant problem, and the sufferer feels trapped.

Definitions of eating disorders (DSM IV, 1994)

Anorexia nervosa

- The refusal to maintain a body weight over a minimum normal weight for age and height (i.e. weight loss leading to body weight 15 per cent below that expected) or failure to make the expected weight gain during a period of growth, leading to a body weight 15 per cent below that expected.
- An intense fear of gaining weight or becoming fat even though underweight.
- A disturbance* in the way in which one's body weight, size or shape is experienced, an undue influence of body shape and weight on self-evaluation, or a denial of the seriousness of low body weight.
- In females, the absence of at least three consecutive menstrual cycles when otherwise expected to occur (primary or secondary amenorrhoea).

*It should be noted that the disturbance does not occur exclusively during episodes of anorexia nervosa.

> **Activity 7.5: If your surgery does not have a good set of weighing scales and a stadiometer (for measuring height), try to persuade the budget holder(s) to purchase some.**

Bulimia nervosa

- Recurrent episodes of binge eating, an episode of binge eating being characterized by both of the following:
  – eating in a discrete period of time (e.g. any 2-hour period) an amount of food that is definitely larger than most people would eat during a similar period of time in similar circumstances;
  – a sense of lack of control over eating during the episode, for example a feeling that one cannot stop or control how much one is eating.

- Recurrent compensatory behaviour in order to prevent weight gain, for example self-induced vomiting, the use of laxatives, the use of other drugs such as diuretics, and fasting or excessive exercise.
- A minimum average of two binge eating and inappropriate compensatory behaviours per week for at least 3 months.
- Self-evaluation that is unduly influenced by body shape and weight.

Binge eating disorder

All the criteria for bulimia nervosa are met except that the compensatory behaviour is absent or infrequent.

It is possible to have a mixture of the features described above, and the sufferer may, in the course of time, move from one eating disorder to another. It is also possible to have some but not all of the features; these are called partial syndromes or defined as eating disorders not otherwise specified (EDNOS). It is thought that these may be more common than the full disorders.

Many mental health services are reluctant to recognize binge eating disorder (BED) as a true eating disorder.

Prevalence

There have been numerous studies that have estimated the prevalence rates of anorexia nervosa (AN) and bulimia nervosa (BN). Wide variations have been reported because of the relative rarity of eating disorders, the reluctance of sufferers to participate in surveys and the fluctuating nature of the illness, the latter posing difficulties in the interpretation of symptoms. 'A General Practitioner's Guide to Eating Disorders' (Myers et al., 1993) estimated that an average general practitioner list that includes 2000 patients at any one time is likely to have:

- 1–2 patients with AN;
- 18 patients with BN;
- 5–10 per cent of adolescent girls who are using weight-reducing techniques other than dieting, i.e. vomiting, laxative or diuretic abuse, or excessive exercising.

An increasing number of people with eating disorders is being identified. The age of onset for AN is around 15–24 years, peaking at 18 years, but it can occur at any age. BN tends to occur slightly later, between the ages of 15 and 45. Ninety per cent of sufferers are female, but an increasing number of men are coming forward for treatment.

At the end of 1997, there were no figures available for BED and few data on male sufferers.

Causes

There is no single cause, but the commonly found contributory factors are summarized in Box 7.7.

Box 7.7: Factors contributing to eating disorders

Life events
Death of a close relative or friend
Illness of a parent – mental or physical
Divorce or separation of parents
Leaving home
Termination of pregnancy
Sexual or physical abuse, or neglect
Ending of a close relationship
Examinations
Bullying or teasing
Onset of menstruation

Cultural/social influences
Fashion industry
Social pressures to be thin and the stigma of being fat

Low self-esteem
Many sufferers feel a lack of self-worth, sometimes to the point of self-loathing

Personality
Perfectionist
Obsessional, e.g. with tidiness, cleanliness and appearance
High (often unrealistic) expectations of achievements
Compliant and quiet child, prior to the onset of the eating disorder

Family
Difficulty in dealing with problems
Excessive concern about body shape, weight or fitness
Alcohol misuse

Presenting symptoms

Although the individual may present for a wide variety of medical conditions, common symptoms relate to the effects of starvation and purging behaviour (Box 7.8).

Box 7.8: Common presenting symptoms of eating disorders

- Marked changes in weight or very low weight
- Gynaecological problems, e.g. amenorrhoea, delayed menarche, infertility, marked changes in menstrual cycle
- Digestive problems (due to starvation and/or purging behaviour), e.g. abdominal pain or cramps, diarrhoea and constipation (may include requests for laxatives)
- Bloating and fluid retention
- Sleeping difficulties, anxiety, changes in personality. Inability to cope at school, college or work

---

Anorexia nervosa

The anorexic is unlikely to come forward and ask for help. As sufferers see it, there is nothing wrong (the eating disorder has cured the problem), so no treatment is necessary. They usually see themselves as being too fat and will be trying to lose more weight. Sufferers are often brought to the attention of the medical services by relatives alarmed at food refusal and weight loss.

When the disorder is well established, the general appearance is one of emaciation. Low weight in recent-onset AN may be less obvious, and the change in weight or the rate of weight loss may be more pertinent. Other symptoms to look for are related to biological adaptations to starvation; these include amenorrhoea, feeling the cold, low blood pressure, tiredness and weakness.

There are many illnesses in which poor appetite and consequently poor food intake may cause severe weight loss. It is important to establish whether there is a deliberate attempt to restrict food intake in order to lose weight before anorexia nervosa can be suspected.

Bulimia nervosa

BN has been described as a secret disorder, and unless the sufferer discloses her problem, it can lie undetected for many years. Outwardly, the person is usually within the normal weight range and trying to follow a healthy lifestyle. She may present at the general practitioner surgery with symptoms related to the purging behaviour, for example abdominal pain, mouth ulcers and oesophagitis. Occasionally, the complaint is of an inability to diet due to compulsive eating (bingeing). Severe vomiting and laxative abuse can lead to major fluid and electrolyte disturbances, which may need emergency treatment. Depression is more common in BN than AN.

Binge eating disorder

Sufferers are usually overweight and binge on large quantities of food in response to emotional stress, for example examinations, loneliness or bullying. This bingeing is a much more compulsive activity than eating for comfort or boredom and has to be distinguished from these. Young people with binge eating disorders are much more likely to be referred to a dietitian or the practice nurse/practice weight-reducing class than to be diagnosed as the sufferer of an eating disorder.

Treatment and outcome

Most sufferers can be treated on an outpatient basis. Only very severe cases will need admission to hospital.

The mainstays of treatment for eating disorders are:

- education about eating disorders;
- counselling and psychotherapy (e.g. cognitive behaviour therapy);
- family therapy (indicated for sufferers under 18 years of age);
- nutritional counselling.

Specialized services and units may also provide a range of other treatments, such as life skills, creative therapies and relaxation programmes.

The sooner the treatment starts after the onset of the eating disorder, the better the outcome. The practice nurse in primary care is well placed to help sufferers and their families, but there is good evidence that treatment must be at the right time as well as appropriate. It is likely that the sufferer will, sooner or later, need to be referred to a specialist service or at least a therapist who has had some experience in dealing with eating disorders. However, there is much that the practice nurse can do to help.

Practice nurse involvement

Engage the patient in treatment

The first step is to help sufferers to *acknowledge* that they have a problem and that it is psychological in origin. This may take a few sessions, but it is time well spent. Many sufferers will deny they have a problem or play down its seriousness so will not be receptive to treatment if it is offered too soon.

The next step is to *educate* the patient (and her family) about eating disorders. Helpful literature and books can be obtained from:

- the Eating Disorders Association;
- MIND;
- local libraries;
- the Family Doctor Series title 'Eating Disorders', which can be bought from chemist shops.

Teaching sufferers about the ill-effects of starving and purging, and their medical consequences (in both the short and long term), is also helpful, as many do not realize the damage that they are doing to themselves.

Encourage them to join the Eating Disorders Association and/or a self-help group (if your area has one). Some people get better on their own once given relevant information.

Activity 7.6: Find out where the nearest self-help group for eating disorders can be found.

The third step is to motivate the patient to *want to recover and make changes*. Treatment involves facing up to the difficulties that the eating disorder has resolved, so can be a long, painful and sometimes frightening experience. Explaining that treatment will involve talking about feelings as well as the eating problems is helpful in preparing them for therapy.

Finally, reassure the patient, but pay special attention to her family: the anxiety generated by them often makes matters worse. Try to help them to concentrate on talking to their relative about problems rather than battling over food.

Identify and correct medical problems

A full medical examination is essential and needs to include:

- anthropometric data, i.e. height, weight, weight changes and calculation of BMI or plotting data on percentile charts;
- biochemistry (urea and electrolyte and blood glucose levels);
- haematology (white cell count and haemoglobin level);
- physical examination, including blood pressure;
- other signs of self-harm, for example alcohol or drug misuse, cutting, suicide attempts or suicidal thoughts.

Monitoring the above is essential, and the following need to be acted upon quickly:

- a very low weight (a BMI less than 15);
- any serious drop in weight (1 kg per week over 8 weeks);
- escalating purging behaviour;
- suicidal intentions.

The death rate from eating disorders is higher than that from any other psychiatric illness.

Drugs such as appetite stimulants or tranquillizers are not an effective treatment for eating disorders. Antidepressants may be helpful in BN if depression is marked, but they rarely help in AN.

Refer

A practice counsellor, with or without the support of a dietitian, may be able to help in many mild cases. More severe and/or complicated cases may need referral for specialist advice.

Referrals out of the practice will depend on the availability of local services, specialist teams and eating disorders units (either NHS or private). Child and adolescent services will accept young people who are still at school, and adult mental health services will be able to assess older sufferers and recommend treatment.

Activity 7.7: Find out what local mental health services have to offer sufferers, and how to refer.

Summary

Eating disorders may go undiagnosed or unrecognized for many years. Effective treatment depends on the patient wanting to get well and recover from the eating disorder. Some people get better without treatment from professionals. Most people with eating disorders will recover, but a small proportion become chronic sufferers or die from the effects of starvation or suicide.

Very low-weight individuals (with a BMI of less than 15) and those with severe electrolyte disturbances will need urgent medical attention, and hospital admission may need to be considered.

Practice nurses may be the first point of contact for sufferers of eating disorders and must be alert to the potential sufferer when asked to advise on weight and diet. A knowledge of local services and methods of referral is essential for ensuring that these patients receive specialist help to reduce morbidity and premature mortality.

References

Allen I (1991) Family Planning and Pregnancy Counselling Projects for Young People. London: Policy Studies Institute.

Ashken IC, Soddy AG (1980) Study of pregnant school age girls. British Journal of Family Planning 6: 77–82.

Barratt J (1997) The cost and availability of healthy food choices in southern Derbyshire. Journal of Human Nutrition and Dietetics 10(1): 63–9.

Children's Act (1989) Working Together. London: HMSO.

Crawley H (1993) The role of breakfast cereals in the diets of 16–17 year old teenagers in Britain. Journal of Human Nutrition and Dietetics 6(3): 205–16.

Department of Education (1994) Education Act 1993. Sex Education in Schools. Circular 5/94.

Department of Education (1997) Excellence in Schools: A White Paper. London: HMSO.

Department of Health (1989a) Dietary Sugars and Human Disease. COMA. Report on Health and Social Subjects No. 37. London: HMSO.

Department of Health (1989b) The Diets of British School Children. Subcommittee on Nutritional Surveillance. COMA. Report on Health and Social Subjects No. 36. London: HMSO.

Department of Health (1991) Dietary Reference Values for Food Energy and Nutrients for the United Kingdom (DRV). Report on Health and Social Subjects No. 41. London: HMSO.

Department of Health (1992) The Health of the Nation: A Strategy for Health in England. London: HMSO.

Department of Health (1994) Nutritional Aspects of Cardiovascular Disease. Report of the COMA Cardiovascular Review Group. Report on Health and Social Subjects No. 46. London: HMSO.

Department of Health (1995a) Nutrition and Physical Activity Task Forces: Obesity. London: HMSO.

Department of Health (1995b) Variations Sub-group of the Chief Medical Officer's Health of the Nation Working Group. London: HMSO.

Department of Health (1998) Our Healthier Nation. A Summary of the Consultation Paper. London: HMSO.

DSM IV (1994) American Psychiatric Institute Diagnostic and Statistical Manual of Mental Disorders, 4th Edn. Washington, DC: APA.

Family Planning Association (1994) Family Planning Today Fourth Quarter: 3.

Frost JJ, Forrest JD (1995) Understanding the impact of effective teenage pregnancy prevention programs. Family Planning Perspectives 27: 188–95.

Gillick v. Wisbeck and W. Norfolk AHA (1985) 3 AllER 402 HL.

Godfrey KM, Redman CWG, Barker DJP, Osmond C (1991) The effect of maternal anaemia and iron deficiency on the ratio of fetal weight to placental weight. British Journal of Obstetrics and Gynaecology 98: 886–91.

Graham A, Green L, Glasier F (1996) Teenagers, knowledge of emergency contraception: questionnaire survey in South East Scotland. British Medical Journal 312: 1567–9.

Hackett AF, Kirby S, Howie M (1997) A national survey of the diet of children aged 13–14 years living in urban areas of the United Kingdom. Journal of Human Nutrition and Dietetics 10(1): 37–51.

Health Education Authority (1992) Tomorrow's Young Adults: 9–15 Year Olds Look at Alcohol, Drugs, Exercise and Smoking. London: HEA.

Health Education Authority (1995) Diet and Health in School Age Children. London: HEA.

Health Education Authority (1997) Changing What You Eat. London: HEA.

Johnson B, Hackett AF (1997) Eating habits of 11–14 yr old schoolchildren living in less affluent areas of Liverpool, UK. Journal of Human Nutrition and Dietetics 10(2): 135–44.

Leather S (1996) The Making of Modern Malnutrition. London: Caroline Walker Trust.

McCance RA, Widdowson EM (1991) Composition of Foods, 5th Edn. Bath: Bath Press.

McCance RA, Widdowson EM (1996) Meat Products and Dishes, 6th Supplement. Bath: Bath Press.

Moynihan PJ, Anderson AJ, Adamson AF, Rugg-Gunn AJ, Appleton DR, Butler TJ (1994) Dietary sources of iron in English adolescents. Journal of Human Nutrition and Dietetics 7(3): 225–31.

Myers S, Davies MP, Treasure J (1993) A General Practitioner's Guide to Eating Disorders. Maudsley Practical Handbook Series No. 2. London: Bethlem & Maudsley NHS Trust.

National Dairy Council (1989) Fact File 5: Nutrition and Teenagers. London: NDC.

National Dairy Council (1992) Fact File 1: Calcium and Health. London: NDC.

National Forum for Coronary Heart Disease Prevention (1993) Food for Children. London: Hamilton House.

Nelson M, Naismith DJ, Burley V, Gatenby S, Geddes N (1990) Nutrient intakes, vitamin–mineral supplementation and intelligence in British schoolchildren. British Journal of Nutrition 64: 13–22.

Nelson M, White J, Rhodes C (1993) Haemoglobin, ferritin, and iron intakes in British children aged 12–14 years: a preliminary investigation. British Journal of Nutrition 70: 147–55.

NHS Centre for Reviews and Dissemination (1997) Preventing and reducing the adverse effects of unintended teeenage pregnancies. Effective Health Care 3(1): 1–12.

Office for National Statistics (1996) Birth Statistics FMI 23. London: HMSO.

Office of Population Censuses and Surveys (1993) Public Health Standard Dataset. London: OPCS.

Ottley C (1997) Childhood activity and diet in prevention of obesity: a review of the evidence. Health Education Journal 56: 313–20.

Passmore S (1997) Dietary patterns in school meals in secondary schools: a case study using data from cafeteria sales in Birmingham. Health Education Journal 56: 241–50.

Peersman G, Oakley A, Oliver S, Thomas J (1996) Reviews of Effectiveness of Sexual Health Promotion Interventions for Young People. University of London: Social Science Research Unit.

Pollitt E (1995) Does breakfast make a difference in school? Journal of the American Dietetic Association 95(10): 1134–9.

Ranjan V (1993) Pregnancy in the under 16's: waking up to the realities. Professional Care of Mother and Child 3(2): 34–5.

Realeat (1997) Realeat Survey 1984–1987. Newport Pagnell: Realeat Survey Office.

Seamark C, Gray D (1997) Like mother, like daughter: a general practice study of maternal influences on teenage pregnancy. British Journal of General Practice 47: 175–6.

SNAGs (1994) School Nutrition Action Groups – SNAGs. Birmingham: Health Education Unit.

Thomas B (1996) Nutrition in Primary Care. Oxford: Blackwell Science Publications.

Wilson F (1980) Antecedents of adolescent pregnancy. Journal of Biosocial Science 14: 17–25.

Winfield J (1995) Targetting teenagers. Practice Nurse 11(2): 139–42.

Winn S, Roker D, Coleman J (1995) Knowledge about puberty and sexual development in 11–16 year old: implications for health and sex education in schools. Educational Studies 21: 187–201.

Woodward DR, Cunning FJ, Ball PJ, Williams HM, Hornsby H, Boon JA (1997) Does television affect teenagers' food choices. Journal of Human Nutrition and Dietetics (6) 229–36.

Further reading

Brownell KD, Fairburn C (Eds) (1995) Eating Disorders and Obesity, A Comprehensive Handbook. New York: Guilford Press.

Buckroyd J (1996) Anorexia and Bulimia – Your Questions Answered. Dorset: Shaftesbury.

Contraception Education Service (1995) Emergency Contraception Information Pack. London: FPA/HEA.

Dana M, Lawrence M (1989) Women's Secret Disorder. A New Understanding of Bulimia. London: Grafton.

Eating Disorders Association (1995) Eating Disorders. A Guide for Primary Care. Norwich: Eating Disorders Association.

Garner DM, Garfinkel PE (1997) Handbook of Treatment for Eating Disorders, 2nd Edn. New York: Guilford Press.

Health Advisory Service (1996) A Review of Services for People with Eating Disorders in the West Midlands. Birmingham: National Health Service Executive.

Health Education Authority (1995) Diet and Health in School Age Children. London: HEA.

Lawrence M, Dana M (1990) Fighting Food. London: Penguin.

NHS Centre for Reviews and Dissemination (1997) Preventing and reducing the adverse effects of unintended teenage pregnancies. Effective Health Care 3(1): 1–12.

Paediatric Group of the British Dietetic Association. Leaflets: Food for the School Year; and Vegetarianism. Available from British Dietetic Association, 7th Floor, Elizabeth House, 22 Suffolk Street, Queensway, Birmingham B1 1LS.

Palmer R (1980) Anorexia Nervosa. London: Penguin.

Palmer RL (1996) Understanding Eating Disorders. Family Doctor Publications/British Medical Association.

Szmukler G, Dare C, Treasure J (Eds) (1995) Handbook of Eating Disorders:

Theory, Treatment and Research. Chichester: John Wiley & Sons.
Thomas B (1994) Manual of Dietetic Practice. Oxford: Blackwell Scientific Publications.
Thomas B (1996) Nutrition in Primary Care. Oxford: Blackwell Science.

Useful addresses

Child Growth Foundation
2 Mayfield Avenue,
London W4 1PW

Eating Disorders Association
First floor, Wensum House,
103 Prince of Wales Road,
Norwich,
Norfolk NR1 1DW

Get Cooking Pack
3rd Floor, 5-11 Worship Street,
London EC2A 2BH

MIND (National Association for Mental Health)
Granta House, 15/19 Broadway,
London E15 4BQ

School Nutrition Action Groups
Health Education Unit,
MEC, 74 Balden Road,
Harborne,
Birmingham B32 2EN
Tel: 0121–428 2262

Chapter 8
Wound management in general practice

Joy Rainey

This chapter uses the example of wound management to relate some of the theoretical issues discussed within the book to practical care within general practice. These issues can be transferred to most clinical scenarios.

Practice nurses, who are often the initial point of contact for wound management in primary care, must have evidence-based knowledge to make a skilled holistic assessment of both the patient and the wound to enable an appropriate cost-effective treatment plan to be devised.

The principles of wound care relate to all wounds, regardless of size or position, and involve promoting healing within an optimum environment using correct materials and methods of application. The range of wounds encountered by the practice nurse will vary greatly, as will the autonomy for treatment allowed within individual general practices. The following information should enable the reader to understand the rationale behind current wound management theories, assess the patient and choose an appropriate dressing/treatment.

Types of wound

A wound is an abnormal break in the skin, the result of cell death or damage. Wounds are often put into different categories or classified, which enables professionals to share information and experiences knowing that they are talking about similar wounds. Wounds can be classified in several ways, but each is unique and, as such, deserves individual care.

A common way of classifying wounds is into those which heal by primary and by secondary intention. Those healing by primary intention are those whose skin edges have been brought together, usually by sutures, clips, steristrips or surgical adhesive. These may be traumatic lacerations or surgical wounds.

Secondary intention describes healing when the skin edges are not brought together; these have to heal by contracting and filling up with granulation tissue. Such wounds include leg ulcers, sites of pressure damage and dirty surgical or traumatic injuries that may become infected if the skin edges are opposed and secured.

Wounds can also be categorized by the type of tissue within the wound:

- The wound is red and granulating.
- The wound is starting to display signs of the formation of new pink epithelial tissue.
- The wound is yellow and sloughing.
- The wound contains black necrotic tissue.
- The wound is green or infected.

These tissue types are discussed in more detail under wound assessment (see also Figures 8.1–8.5).

Wounds can also be classified by depth. This is a common way of describing pressure sores, several different scales existing for this. An example of this type of scale is the UK consensus classification of pressure sore severity (Stirling Scale; Table 8.1) (Reid and Morison, 1994.) Although it is not usual to see pressure sores in the general

Table 8.1: The UK Consensus classification of pressure sores

Stage	Findings
Stage 1	Discolouration of intact skin (light finger pressure applied to intact skin does not alter the discolouration)
Stage 2	Partial thickness skin loss or damage involving epidermis and/or dermis
Stage 3	Full-thickness skin loss involving damage to or necrosis of subcutaneous tissue but not extending to underlying bone, tendon or joint capsule
Stage 4	Full-thickness skin loss with extensive destruction and tissue necrosis extending to underlying bone, tendon or joint capsule

practitioner's surgery, this type of classification by depth can be used or adapted to describe other wounds.

Although these are the most common ways of categorizing wounds, other methods can be used, including by cause or by the stage of the healing process that the wound has reached.

The healing process

As previously mentioned, wounds can be described as healing by primary or by secondary intention. Healing by primary intention should be achieved for all incised surgical wounds and primary sutured lacerations. Wound healing should be rapid because there is no tissue loss and the skin edges are held together.

In wounds healing by secondary intention, the wound edges are apart and the defect will need to fill with granulation tissue before new epidermis can cover the wound. Such wounds include leg ulcers, open incisions, for example after drainage of an abscess when closure may encourage infection, and full-thickness burns.

Occasionally, wounds are described as healing by tertiary intention. This is desirable if a wound such as a laceration has been contaminated, for example with dirt following an accident. The wound is initially cleaned and left open; if there appears to be little risk of infection, it is then closed in the normal way (Dealey, 1994).

Wound healing is usually described in four physiological phases: the inflammatory, destructive, proliferative and maturation phases (Nursing Times, 1994). In reality, it is a continuous process, the stages merging and overlapping.

Inflammatory stage (0–3 days)

When tissue is injured or disrupted, the body's immediate response is to re-establish haemostasis. Damaged cells and blood vessels release histamine, causing vasodilatation of the surrounding capillaries, which takes serous exudate and white cells to the area of damage (Figure 8.1). It is this increased blood flow and serous exudate that cause local oedema, redness and heat, giving rise to an inflamed appearance.

The coagulation system and platelets cause the blood to clot, which prevents further bleeding or loss of body fluid. Injured vessels thrombose, and red cells become entangled in a fibrin mesh, which begins to dry and become a scab, which is the body's natural defence to keep out micro-organisms. Phagocytic white cells (polymorphs

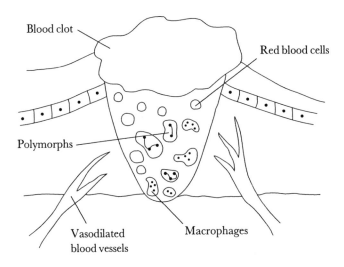

Figure 8.1: Inflammatory stage: 0–3 days.

and macrophages) are attracted to the area to defend against bacteria, ingest debris and begin the process of repair. In a clean acute wound, this stage lasts up to three days; if the wound is infected or necrotic tissue is present, this stage is prolonged.

Destructive phase (1–6 days)

White cells line the walls of blood vessels and migrate through the walls, which become more porous, into the surrounding tissue. Here phagocytic cells break down devitalized necrotic tissue, and the macrophages engulf and ingest bacteria and dead tissue. In addition, macrophages stimulate the development of new blood vessels and the formation and multiplication of fibroblasts (Figure 8.2, page 258), which are in turn responsible for the synthesis of collagen and other connective tissue. This stage normally lasts 1–6 days, but white cell activity can be compromised in dry, exposed wounds (Morison, 1992).

Proliferative phase (3–24 days)

The fibroblasts continue to multiply, producing collagen fibrils, which form a fibrous network (Figure 8.3). This traps red blood cells, which go on to become involved in new capillary loops. At this stage, the tissue is very delicate, having none of the organization of normal tissue. This granulation tissue is so called because of its red granular appearance.

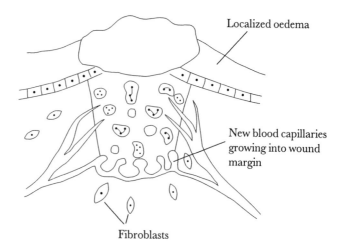

Figure 8.2: Destructive/migratory phase: 1–6 days.

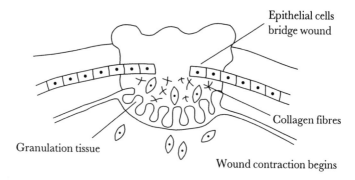

Figure 8.3: Proliferation/granulation stage: 3–24 days.

As the collagen matures, there is a rapid increase in tensile strength. Signs of inflammation subside and the process of contraction begins. In an open wound this stage may be prolonged because more collagen is needed to repair the tissue defect.

Maturation phase (24 days – 1 year)

When the wound has filled with granulation tissue, the collagen fibres pull on the wound, causing it to contract and become smaller. This speeds up the healing process as less collagen will be necessary to repair the defect. As the wound space decreases, vascularity also decreases, fibroblasts shrink and collagen fibres change the red granulation tissue to white avascular tissue as epithelium migrates inward (Figure 8.4).

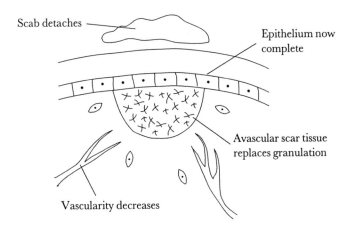

Scab detaches

Epithelium now complete

Avascular scar tissue replaces granulation

Vascularity decreases

Figure 8.4: Maturation stage: 24 days–1 year.

Epithelial cells migrate from the wound edge, sweat glands and the remnants of hair follicles. They migrate over the granulation tissue until they meet with like cells from another area of the wound, sometimes forming islands in the wound centre. This process is slowed down if the wound is dry and is covered by a scab (or eschar). In this case, they have to burrow under the dry scab (see moist wound healing, below). Migrating cells lose their ability to divide, so epithelialization depends on the ability of like cells to keep meeting. When the surface is covered with epithelial cells, the epithelium thins. Hair follicles are not replaced. Wound maturation usually takes between 24 days and one year.

Moist wound healing

Wound care management has traditionally encouraged nurses to allow wounds to dry out and form a scab. This was thought to provide a mechanical barrier to infection and be the most appropriate treatment. Extensive research has shown that this is not the case, although some clinicians and many patients still cling to traditional methods.

Work on moist wound healing started in the early 1960s. The most quoted research in relation to this is that of Winter (1962), who conducted a clinical trial using superficial wounds on pigs. Half of these wounds were allowed to dry out and form scabs, whilst the other half were covered with polythene, thus creating a moist environment. The results showed that those covered with polythene epithelialized nearly twice as fast as those wounds allowed to dry out. After examining the histology, Winter concluded that, in the dry wounds, epithelial cells were handicapped when migrating across the wound surface by the collagen fibres joining the scab to the surface of the wound. Epithelial cells in the moist wounds could migrate more quickly through the wound exudate and did not need to traverse a scabbed area. Dyson et al. (1988) have shown that a moist wound moves through the inflammatory stage of healing more quickly than a dry wound and produces greater capillary growth.

It was initially thought that the moist environment might encourage greater bacterial growth and lead to a higher number of wound infections, but this view has been disproved. Studies by Hutchinson and Lawrence (1991) showed that the reverse was true and that occluded wounds showed a lower rate of infection.

Since the late 1970s, manufacturing companies have been creating dressings that give a moist environment to speed wound healing. Some clinicians who still cling to traditional products such as gauze use the higher unit cost of modern products as a reason to support their choice. However, modern products encourage wounds to heal faster and become infected less often. The unit cost of each dressing becomes less relevant when viewed in relation to patient discomfort, nursing time and the greater use of other materials (e.g. sterile gloves, aprons and dressing packs) and antibiotics.

Wound assessment

Wound assessment is commonly a responsibility left to the nurse. In order for the care given to be appropriate, it is important that assessment is carried out thoroughly to identify a goal of treatment, for example to protect and keep moist, the most appropriate treatment is then chosen and the treatment is evaluated to check for progress or deterioration.

It is also important that this assessment and any subsequent evaluations are clearly documented, for several reasons. First, it allows evaluation to take place. If good records are not kept, the evaluation is likely to be vague and subjective, relying on comments such as 'looking better' or 'healing well', which tell us nothing about the state of the wound. This is perhaps even more important if more than one person is responsible for the patient's care. Second, records are of extreme importance in case of complaint or litigation. In legal terms, if it is not recorded, the care was not carried out, so records must be timely, accurate and clear (see Chapter 1).

Although assessment might seem to be a lengthy process, time spent assessing a wound should lead to the selection of appropriate treatment. This should optimize wound healing and lead to a swifter resolution of care (see Chapter 2).

> **Activity 8.1: Take out some records you made about a patient's wound from three years ago. What do these records tell you about the wound's appearance, progress and history? Can you recall this wound with any clarity or detail? Would you be happy to stand in court and defend your practice, relying on the records you have made?**

Thorough assessment of the wound will take time, but, if it leads to the correct treatment being chosen with optimized wound healing, it is time well spent. In the longer term, the patient requires fewer episodes of care. Assessment details can be written in the patient's notes or on a purpose-made chart (Figure 8.5 page 262). The following guidelines suggest areas to include.

Wound type

It is important that the type or cause of the wound is identified and recorded. Personal observation suggests that acute wounds such as lacerations, bites and post-operative wounds are usually clearly identified but that chronic wounds such as leg ulcers are generalized. It is important that the exact underlying causes are identified: Is it a venous ulcer? Is it an arterial ulcer? Is it a malignancy? Did the wound start from trauma or a bite, in which case there may be no underlying disease?

The treatment of each wound type is different, and in the case of venous and arterial ulcers opposite, so without identification, the chosen treatment may be incorrect. (Leg ulcers will be discussed in more detail below.)

Position of the wound

This should be clearly documented and may be aided by the use of diagrams. The position of leg ulcers can also aid diagnosis.

Size of the wound

This should be recorded so that healing or deterioration can be observed. Both the nurse and the patient can be motivated if healing can be observed. This also encourages patient compliance to

Patient name .... Position of wound ....

Type of wound .... Duration of wound ....

Date						
Size of wound Max. width Max. length						
Type of tissue within wound e.g. slough, necrotic, granulation tissue						
Exudate Amount, colour?						
Odour None, some, offensive?						
Pain When, where, severity?						
Surrounding skin Erythema, wet/dry eczema						
Infection Suspected, swab taken, result?						
Treatment summary: Cleansing lotion Topical treatment of wound and surrounding skin Primary dressing Secondary dressing Fixed by						
Assessed by						

Figure 8.5: Example of a wound assessment form.

continue with treatment not met with enthusiasism, such as compression therapy.

The simplest way to record wound size is to take the maximum dimensions with a ruler (Figure 8.6). A more accurate way is to trace the wound, using either a purpose-made chart (available from several dressing manufacturing companies), acetate sheets or the clear packaging in which many dressings come. The tracing can be either stored in the patient's notes as it is or used as a template to draw round in the notes. Consider whether or not the plastic is sterile. It is advisable to hold non-sterile materials slightly above the wound surface or to cleanse the surface touching the wound both before and after use with an Alcowipe.

Photographs are the most accurate way of recording the size and appearance of large wounds. If using personal cameras for this purpose, be aware of where the film is to developed with regard to patient confidentiality. Some developers have films on display in shop windows, and postal services can go astray. A Polaroid camera is useful to obtain instant pictures. Try to keep the background plain so that the patient's limb and wound stand out. It is also useful to attach a piece of tape on which the date and the patient's name or initials are written; this helps to identify photographs or check their chronological order.

The depth of the wound is more difficult to measure, but using a sterile probe is probably the most accurate method. These are sometimes available from pharmaceutical companies.

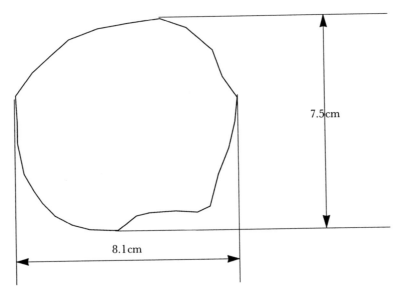

7.5cm

8.1cm

Figure 8.6: Measuring a wound.

History of the wound

It is worth asking how long the wound has been present, who until now has being dressing it and what treatments have already been used. This will give some indication of any allergies or treatments that have previously failed. The wound may be a recurrence of a leg ulcer (particularly venous), and the treatment of previous episodes of ulceration may be relevant.

Surrounding skin

It is important to assess the surrounding skin. Any redness or erythema may indicate infection. If the patient has fragile skin, perhaps caused by medication such as long-term steroid use, it may be inappropriate to apply an adhesive dressing.

Leg ulcers may be surrounded by varicose eczema, which may require an emollient, or by contact dermatitis from previous treatments, which may require a short course of a topical steroid cream.

Tissue within the wound

The state of the tissue within the wound will help to identify the goal of treatment and in many ways identify an appropriate treatment. There may be more than one type of tissue within the wound, in which case an estimate of the percentage of each type should be made, for example 70 per cent granulation and 30 per cent slough.

The wound may contain black or necrotic tissue, which is the result of tissue death secondary to ischaemia. It may be soft and spongy or form a hard eschar over the surface of the wound. This will always delay healing and increase the chances of wound infection.

The aim of treatment is debridement by use of an appropriate dressing, or, if necessary, a surgical opinion on sharp debridement can be sought.

The yellow or sloughy tissue formed in many chronic wounds is made up of dead cells and serous exudate. This needs to be removed to optimize healing and is a similar process to debridement. It is important not to mistake exposed tendons or epithelial islands for slough as they may have a similar appearance.

Red or granulating wounds have fragile new tissue forming, which is easily damaged. The aim of treatment is to protect the tissue and provide a moist environment to optimize healing. Particular care should be taken during wound cleansing, and a dressing should be selected that will not adhere to the surface of the wound and cause trauma during dressing changes.

Pink or epithelial tissue is the new layer of epidermis that will cover the wound once it has filled with granulation tissue. The epithelial cells that migrate from the wound margins sometimes meet to form clusters or islands on the wound surface. The movement of these cells is aided by a moist environment, so the chosen dressing should again provide this environment and protect the wound surface.

Infected tissue within the wound often has a greenish appearance. The routine swabbing of wounds is inappropriate for the diagnosis of infection and is an unnecessary cost. It is important to understand that wounds may have transient organisms present that swab results detect in small numbers. These organisms are often the usual skin flora and are not usually regarded as pathogenic.

Many chronic wounds become colonized by a variety of bacteria that may be potentially pathogenic. 'Colonization' refers to organisms that have multiplied and are often present in high numbers, but infection is not inevitable, and many colonized wounds heal without problems. These micro-organisms can, however, be dispersed during dressing changes, and measures should be taken to limit this.

Wound infection occurs when colonizing bacteria reach sufficient numbers to cause distinct clinical signs. These include erythema, oedema, increased exudate, offensive odour, pain and pyrexia (Thompson and Smith, 1994). If a wound exhibits one or more of these signs, it is appropriate to take a wound swab. Immunocompromised or diabetic patients may fail to show signs of inflammation or clinical infection; this may require a wound swab to be taken if the wound is failing to respond to treatment, even if the usual clinical signs are not present.

Occasionally, other patients do not exhibit the classic immune response (Plewa, 1990). If wounds fail to respond to treatment, it is worth considering the seven other criteria that may indicate infection (Box 8.1).

There is some controversy over the best method of performing a wound swab. Cooper and Lawrence (1996) suggest gentle irrigation of the wound with normal saline, and swabbing in a zigzag motion over the entire wound surface while slowly rotating the swab.

The treatment of infection should be by systemic antibiotics. The use of topical treatment with antibacterial creams can lead to the growth of resistant organisms (Morgan, 1987) and should be avoided.

> **Box 8.1: Criteria that may indicate infection (Cutting and Harding, 1994)**
>
> - Delayed healing
> - Discolouration
> - Friable granulation tissue that bleeds easily
> - Unexpected tenderness
> - Pocketing at the base of the wound
> - Bridging of soft tissue and epithelium
> - Wound breakdown

Pain

The patient's level of pain should be assessed and treated with appropriate analgesia. Other factors to consider are:

- Is the pain ischaemic? (If the leg ulcer is arterial in origin, a vascular opinion may be appropriate – see below.)
- Is the wound infected?
- Is the dressing causing pain either by drying and adhering to the wound surface, or by causing an allergic reaction?
- Is the wound painful at dressing change because the dressing has dried out or is being removed inappropriately?

Wound odour

Wound odour can be very distressing for the patient, often occurring in heavily infected or fungating wounds. Personal experience shows that this may be one reason for a patient seeking treatment. Some dressings may cause odour when they interact with wound exudate; if this is expected to happen, either at dressing change or if the dressing leaks, it is worth warning the patient not to worry that the wound has become infected.

Charcoal dressings should be used if available. Oral or topical metronidazole may reduce odour (Newman et al., 1989), and aromatherapy oils may be applied to the outer dressing to mask the odour.

General assessment of the patient – factors affecting healing

As well as assessing the wound itself, it is important to look at the patient holistically. Many factors, some of which are listed in Box 8.2,

---

Box 8.2: Factors affecting healing

- Age
- Concurrent disease
- Nutritional status
- Drugs
- Smoking
- Excessive alcohol consumption

---

influence wound healing. If these are not addressed, healing will be delayed or may even fail to take place. Not all of the factors can be treated, but if they are highlighted, one can at least gain an understanding of why healing is slow.

Age

As people age, their metabolic processes slow down, which prolongs tissue repair. Wound infection may also be more common as immunocompetence becomes less specific and inflammation less effective (David, 1986). The elderly are more likely to have chronic concurrent illness that may delay healing and to require drug therapy.

Concurrent disease

Diabetes has long been associated with poor wound healing, so it is important to control diabetes if wound healing is to be achieved. Diabetics are also more susceptible to wound infection.

Cardiovascular and pulmonary disease may also delay wound healing because the transport of oxygen to the wound site may be inadequate, and oxygen is essential for wound healing.

Uraemia increases the risk of wound dehiscence because of a reduction in collagen deposition. Granulation may also be delayed.

Thyroid or pituitary deficiency may also delay healing as a result of slowed metabolic rates. Cushing's syndrome treated with steroids will also delay healing.

Nutritional status

Both obesity and malnourishment inhibit wound healing. Gross obesity is likely to make the patient less mobile, thus leading to venous stasis. Adipose tissue is also poorly oxygenated. Advice from a community dietitian may be needed in some cases.

Poor nutrition and malnourishment adversely affect wound healing in many ways. The links between nutrients and healing are shown in Table 8.2. It should be remembered that injury may also lead to a patient's energy demands being higher than usual, and that protein is also lost in wound exudate.

Table 8.2: Important nutrients in wound healing

Nutrient	Role
Protein	Repair and replacement of tissue Energy
Carbohydrate	Energy Spares protein for wound healing
Vitamin C	Collagen synthesis Immunity
Vitamin B12	Protein synthesis
Zinc	Tissue repair Protein synthesis
Iron	Haemoglobin production

If a patient is unable to maintain a good nutritional status, dietary supplements may be necessary, either in the form of tablets (for example, zinc supplements and multivitamins), by injection (for example, Neocytamen and iron) or as meal replacements or supplements.

Drug therapy

Drugs taken therapeutically for other conditions may inhibit wound healing.

Anti-inflammatory drugs, both steroidal and non-steroidal, will delay wound healing and are commonly used to treat arthritis, which is often a problem in the elderly. Aspirin, commonly self-administered or given to treat circulatory disease, will have the same effect. These drugs are designed to suppress inflammation, which is essential for tissue repair.

Immunosuppressive drugs inhibit white cell activity and thus delay the clearance of wound debris. Patients on these drugs are at a high risk of developing a wound infection and may require prophylactic antimicrobial therapy and careful monitoring. Thought needs to be given to timing appointments for these patients in order to reduce the risks of cross-infection (see Chapter 3).

Cytotoxic drugs arrest cell division and also reduce protein production. This is true for both malignant cells and those vital for tissue repair.

Smoking

Smoking alters platelet function, leading to a higher risk of blood clots blocking smaller vessels. Smokers also have reduced haemoglobin function (David, 1986). This means that less haemoglobin is available for oxygen transport, thus adversely affecting wound healing. The risk of arterial disease is increased, which may cause tissue ischaemia and necrosis.

Alcohol

Patients who are heavy drinkers may have liver disease, which can result in a reduction in the number of platelets and clotting factors. They may also have a lower resistance to infection. Gastritis and diarrhoea may also predispose to malnourishment through malabsorption and anaemia caused by blood loss.

Wound cleansing

It is generally accepted that cleansing wounds by swabbing with cotton wool or gauze results in these materials shedding fibres into the wound; these may act as a focus for infection (Draper, 1985). Despite this knowledge, dressing packs available on the drug tariff all contain cotton wool, which should be discarded. Vigorous swabbing may also damage healthy tissue. Irrigation is therefore generally the preferred method.

Which wounds will benefit from cleansing?

Traumatic wounds that contain particles of dirt or other matter will benefit from vigorous irrigation (Lawrence, 1997). Wounds may also benefit from cleansing to remove gross exudate, the remains of previous topical applications and crusting (Miller and Dyson, 1996; Lawrence, 1997), although research suggests that cleansing to remove bacteria is ineffective (Miller and Dyson, 1996): bacteria are not removed but merely redistributed around the wound surface. It is pointless to cleanse wounds routinely, this being appropriate only for removing debris or old dressing material. Reasons for not cleansing should be explained to the patient to avoid any misunderstandings, because most patients think that cleansing is essential.

What fluid should be used for wound cleansing?

The most frequently used fluids are antiseptics, tap water and sterile saline.

Antiseptics

There is little evidence to suggest that the use of antiseptics reduces the bacterial content of wounds, and wounds do not need to be sterile to heal. Current thinking suggests that the use of antiseptics is not advantageous in optimizing wound healing. Miller and Dyson (1996) list some of the criticisms levied against antiseptics:

- Antiseptics do not come into contact with bacteria long enough to kill them during normal wound cleansing.
- Bacteria may become resistant to antiseptics, and those antiseptics containing cetrimide or chlorhexidine may grow bacteria under certain conditions.
- The frequent use of antiseptics may contribute towards bacterial resistance to antibiotics, although there is as yet no proven link.
- Antiseptics adversely affect blood flow in the healing wound.
- Antiseptics are inactivated by organic matter such as pus and wound exudate.

If an antiseptic is to be used, the following are suggested by Lawrence (1997) to be the safer options:

- Chlorhexidine – this is a good skin and hard surface disinfectant and shows low toxicity to living tissue in animal models.
- Povidone iodine – iodine kills bacteria rapidly, possibly within a few seconds, but can impair the microcirculation in animals.

Tap water

One study conducted with tap water found that there was less infection in wounds cleansed with tap water, and no bacteria were transferred to the wound (Angeras et al., 1991). However, some cell damage may occur as a result of lowered osmotic pressure, and this may result in pain (Lawrence, 1997).

Sterile normal saline

Saline in a 0.9 per cent solution has an osmotic pressure similar to that found in tissue in mammals. This reinforces the fact that saline baths are inappropriate because the concentrations vary widely. Saline is currently favoured as the treatment of choice, minimizing the risk of tissue damage and pain. It should be used as a warm solution (see below).

The ideal dressing

Several criteria have been suggested for the ideal dressing (Morgan, 1987). The most important will be discussed and their implications for nursing practice highlighted; others will be listed.

The dressing should provide a moist environment

A primary factor in optimizing healing is that the dressing should provide a moist environment (see above). All of the modern occlusive dressings should provide this type of environment.

Nursing implication

No dry dressings should be used on open wounds because these will allow the area to dry out and thus impede healing.

The wound should be kept free from excess exudate

Although the wound needs to be kept moist, it must not become wet. This causes the surrounding skin to become soggy and macerated, and may lead to further tissue breakdown.

Nursing implication

A dressing should be selected that provides the correct amount of absorbency. All dressings are designed with particular types of wound in mind; for example, alginates are designed for highly exuding wounds, and vapour-permeable films for wounds with very little exudate. This is an important criterion in dressing selection.

The dressing should provide thermal insulation

Wound healing is optimized when wounds are kept at body temperature. If the temperature of the wound drops, mitotic activity slows down, thus delaying wound healing. Leukocytic activity and oxyhaemaglobin dissociation are also disrupted by a drop in wound temperature (Thomas, 1990; Miller and Dyson, 1996).

Nursing implication

Lock (1980) and Myers (1982) found that, after cleansing, it could take a wound up to 40 minutes to regain body temperature, and a further three hours for mitotic activity to return to normal. Thus it is advisable to warm the saline prior to wound cleansing, to keep wounds exposed for a short a time as possible, to try not to disturb wounds unnecessarily and to consider the type of material being used; for example, cotton gauze will keep a wound at around 27°C, whereas a hydrocolloid or foam dressing will increase the temperature to 35°C (Thomas, 1990).

The dressing should be impermeable to micro-organisms

This should work in both directioins. Whilst micro-organisms should be kept away from wounds, it is also undesirable to have micro-organisms from a wound spreading to the environment.

Nursing implication

Any non-adhesive dressing should be taped 'like a picture frame' if the surrounding skin is in good condition, or bandaged to cover the dressing completely. If 'strike-through' occurs, a warm, wet passage for micro-organisms is created, and secondary padding should be applied or the wound redressed.

The dressing should be free from particulate contaminants

Modern dressings are designed to high standards and will not shed fibres or contaminants on to the wound surface. However, traditional gauze, lint or cotton wool may shed fibres that can serve as a focus for infection.

Nursing implication

No dry dressings that shed should be used on open wounds.

The dressing should not cause trauma to the wound

If the chosen dressing adheres to the wound, trauma and pain may occur when the dressing is removed. The ideal healing environment should be free from materials that adhere; this is provided by all modern dressings.

Nursing implication

Traditional dressings such as cotton gauze and paraffin gauze should not be used on open wounds. Adherence occurs as the wound exudate becomes incorporated into the gauze and dries out, adhering to the tissue below. Removal causes the top layer of granulation tissue to be removed with the dressing. Paraffin gauze leaves a criss-cross pattern where new granulation tissue has grown through the mesh, illustrating the pattern quite graphically.

The dressing should allow gaseous exchange

This is a complex issue. It has been noted that angiogenesis (the formation of new blood vessels) in granulating wounds takes place rapidly in the hypoxic environment of occlusive dressings such as hydrocolloids (Cherry and Ryan, 1985). However, when a wound begins to show signs of new epidermis forming, this appears more effectively in a more oxygen-rich environment (Silver, 1985).

Nursing implication

It may be appropriate to use an occlusive dressing when a wound needs to granulate but better to switch to an oxygen-permeable dressing (for example, a foam dressing) to encourage granulation.

The dressing should be available

Is the dressing available to community nurses? Is it a prescribable product? If not, how will you access it?

Nursing implication

Many nurses have arrangements in which they order one item from the pharmacist and exchange it for something of the same value. This is illegal. Even though it is done with the patient's best interest at heart, this action constitutes fraud; if prosecuted, the nurse could face a fine, imprisonment and dismissal.

Activity 8.2: Consider the following list and decide what implications these have for your practice. Once you have reached the end of the list, decide which of the criteria you feel are the most important. The dressing should:

- be safe to use, i.e. practice should be research based;
- be acceptable to the patient;
- be cost-effective – do not think simply in terms of unit cost;
- be capable of standardization and evaluation;
- allow monitoring of the wound;
- provide mechanical protection;
- be non-flammable;
- be sterilizable;
- be conformable and mouldable;
- require infrequent changing.

At the time of writing, no one dressing meets all these criteria. It is therefore important to assess the wound thoroughly, decide on a treatment goal and select the most appropriate dressing from those available.

Dressing types

Many types of wound dressing are now available, and it can be difficult to choose the one most appropriate to the wound. This section attempts to place the dressings into broad categories, giving some suggestions for their appropriate use. The dressings mentioned are not the only ones available, and further information can be obtained from a text such as the 'Formulary of Wound Management Products' (Morgan, 1994).

For information about methods of application, time between dressing changes, removal and contraindications, see the manufacturers' instructions. Only dressings available on the drug tariff are discussed.

Alginate dressings

These dressings are made from seaweed, which contains large quantities of alginate. They are highly absorbent so should not be used on wounds with very little exudate because they will adhere to the wound surface. Some clinicians wet the dressing with saline, but this seems pointless as the dressing is designed to be highly absorbent.

All alginates are highly absorbent and form a gel on contact with wound exudate, giving a moist environment whilst absorbing excess fluid. They may be used on flat wounds and also to pack cavity wounds. Some are manufactured as ropes and ribbons specifically for this purpose but are not available on drug tariff. A secondary dressing is required.

Examples of alginates are Kaltostat (Convatec), Kaltogel (Convatec), Seasorb (Coloplast), Sorbsan (Pharma-Plast), Sorbsan Plus (Pharma-Plast) and Tegagel (3M).

Bead dressings

These dressings are made up of polysaccharide beads. They are indicated for wet, sloughy wounds and should not be used on clean or dry wounds. The beads are extremely hydrophilic and will cause pain if the wound is too dry. Debrisan (Kabi Pharmacia) is available as beads, paste or absorbent pads. Iodosorb and Iodoflex (Perstorp Pharma) both contain iodine and have been used with some success on wounds with superficial infection or superficial wounds contaminated with multi-resistant *Staphylococcus aureus*. All require a secondary dressing.

Enzyme dressings

Varidase (Wyeth Laboratories) is a dry powder containing two enzymes: streptokinase and streptodornase. Varidase is designed to debride necrotic or very sloughy wounds. It can be reconstituted with sterile saline and applied as a soak to dry scabs that have been cross-hatched with a scapel; some practitioners inject under scabs, but this must be done with care so that healthy tissue is not affected. An alternative is to reconstitute the powder with 5 ml sterile water and mix it with 15 ml intrasite gel. Whichever method of application is chosen, a secondary dressing is required. When mixing Varidase powder with any solution, care must be taken not to shake the vial vigorously or the enzymes will become denatured and the treatment ineffective. All patients treated with Varidase show an increase in antistreptokinase titre (Morgan, 1994), so it would seem sensible not to use it on patients at risk of myocardial infarction.

Foam dressings (including hydropolymer and hydrocellular dressings)

Foam dressings are generally highly absorbent and create a moist environment for wound healing; they can be used on a wide variety of wounds. They are available without adhesive, which is useful if the surrounding skin is damaged or fragile, or as adhesive dressings. They can be used on their own or as a secondary dressing, for example with hydogels.

Non-adhesive foams include Allevyn (Smith & Nephew), Lyofoam (Seton) and Lyofoam Extra (Seton). Lyofoam is also useful for resolving overgranulation. Adhesive foams include Allevyn Adhesive (Smith & Nephew), Combiderm (Convatec), Spyrosorb (Perstorp Pharma) and Tielle (Johnson & Johnson).

Hydrogels

Amorphous gels have a high water content. They are very useful for debriding or desloughing wounds by rehydrating the dead tissue, thus allowing the body to shed this tissue by autolysis. Gels are designed to be used on sloughy or necrotic wounds with a low-to-medium amount of exudate, but can also be used on flat wounds and to fill cavities. They are also reported to reduce pain at the wound site (Morgan, 1994). They require a secondary dressing.

Examples of hydrogels are Intrasite gel (Smith & Nephew), Nugel (Johnson & Johnson) and Sterigel (Seton).

Hydrocolloid dressings

Hydrocolloid dressings made from combinations of synthetic polymers are one of the oldest of the 'modern' products and are used in many situations. They are waterproof, adhesive, interactive dressings that form a gel on contact with wound exudate. This may have a slight odour, which is normal. Hydrocolloids can aid desloughing and can be used on wounds with a light-to-medium exudate. Their occlusive nature provides a hypoxic environment that stimulates angiogenisis (Cherry and Ryan, 1985), and the moist environment gives pain relief by keeping nerve endings moist (Morgan, 1994).

Examples of hydrocolloids are Comfeel (Coloplast), Granuflex (Convatec) and Tegasorb (3M). Extra-thin versions are also available as Comfeel Transparent (Coloplast) and Duoderm (Convatec). All the hydrocolloids can be used alone or as a secondary dressing (manufacturers' recommendations should be checked).

Hydrocolloid gel dressings

Granugel (Convatec) is a gel that contains hydrocolloid for desloughing and debriding wounds, and can also be applied to clean wounds. It requires a secondary dressing such as Granuflex.

Vapour-permeable film dressings

These were the first type of modern dressing to be produced. Waterproof, adhesive films create a moist environment but have no fluid-handling capabilities. They can be used on superficial wounds with minimal exudate, prophylactically (for example to reduce shearing forces), on wounds healing by primary intention, or as secondary dressings securing other products.

Examples of film dressings are Bioclusive (Johnson & Johnson), Epiview (Convatec), Opsite flexigrid (Smith & Nephew) and Tegaderm (3M).

Treatment of minor traumatic wounds

Patients may present at a general practice with a variety of minor injuries rather than attending the accident and emergency department. It is important that when there is any doubt about underlying damage, the patient is advised to attend casualty.

Wounds that have been caused accidentally are likely to be contaminated with dirt or bacteria. In addition to having his wound treated, the patient will need advice about tetanus cover and any antibiotic therapy that may be required, for example following a dog bite. Wounds should be thoroughly irrigated with warmed normal saline to remove as much dirt and contamination as possible.

If a wound has been caused, for example, by glass or metal, it is important to ensure that no fragments remain. Grazes often contain grit and grime, which must be removed to avoid a tattooing effect when the graze has healed. If the patient requires the removal of foreign bodies, he or she should be advised either to see the general practitioner or to go to accident and emergency.

Once the wound is clean, it is important to decide whether it is possible to close it. Larger wounds, wounds to the face or those over a joint may require suturing, either within the surgery or in the accident and emergency department.

Smaller lacerations may be held together with reinforced tape such as steristrips. The skin edges should be brought together as closely as possible. Ensure that the skin is dry, and place the first tape in the centre of the wound. Use further closures to oppose the sides of the wound, and then place further ones in any gaps to give a neat finish. Cover with a non-adherent dressing and remove in 5–7 days.

Surgical glue can be useful in managing some straight wounds, especially in children. Application is less traumatic for the child, who will not require local anaesthetic or sutures, and it also reduces medical and nursing time. Refer to the manufacturer's instructions for application.

Small scalp wounds may be closed by tying the hairs from either side of the wound, which prevents shaving the area and gives a neat scar (David, 1986).

Pretibial lacerations are common in the elderly, who have very fragile skin, so great care must be taken if an adhesive dressing is chosen in order to ensure that no further skin tears are made. A skin flap may be taped back into place, but is often too thin to be viable as there will be a poor blood supply to the superficial tissue. In this case, trimming the flap is an option, allowing the wound to heal by secondary intention. Problems arising from these injuries are important in patients with vascular changes: a poor arterial blood supply may delay wound healing, and problems with the venous circulation may result in a venous ulcer.

Small burns and scalds may be seen. Any burn of significant size, of full thickness or over a joint should be referred to accident and emergency. The initial treatment is to cool the surface of the burn or scald with cold water for a minimum of 10 minutes or until it no longer hurts. Blisters often form, and if intact should be left, as micro-organisms cannot enter intact skin. Where blisters have ruptured, how the wound should be treated will depend on the state of the tissue. The wound can be initially treated with flamazine, paraffin gauze, a non-adherent dressing and padding, reviewed after one day and assessed for treatment as wound needs dictate.

Treatment of post-operative wounds

Surgical wounds are usually closed with sutures or clips, which are left in place for between five and seven days depending on the type of surgery and the depth of the wound they are closing.

Studies have shown that after 24 hours the skin will have formed a natural barrier at the suture or clip line, which means that a dressing may be unnecessary (Chrintz, 1989). Patients will require dressings if there is any leakage from the suture line or as a protection against friction from clothing. Certain areas, such as the groin following varicose vein surgery, may be particularly prone to friction and may require a light dressing to absorb any perspiration and reduce friction. Because the skin edges have been brought together, traditional dressings such as gauze or melonin are often used, although these may not be comfortable and are not waterproof (Miller, 1995). It may be appropriate to consider a more modern alternative such as a semi-permeable film dressing, a polyurethane dressing or a thin hydrocolloid. The advantages of these dressings include (Thomas, 1990):

- comfort;
- less bulk;
- the fact that they do not require bandaging or taping into position;
- that they are waterproof;
- that they can, in most cases, be left in position until the sutures or clips can be removed.

Once the sutures or clips have been removed, a dressing should not be necessary unless the wound continues to exude from any areas along the suture line.

Treatment of leg ulcers

The management of patients with leg ulceration is a problem commonly encountered by community nurses. Studies have shown that between 65 per cent and 85 per cent of these cases are managed exclusively by the primary health care team (Kendrick et al., 1994). This care is costly. In 1990, the leg ulcer service from Charing Cross Hospital, London, estimated the annual cost of treating a leg ulcer to be between £2700 and £5200 per patient. This suggests that the treatment of leg ulcers costs the NHS between £300 million and £600 million annually for the UK as a whole (Morison, 1991).

A leg ulcer can be defined as an area of discontinuity of the epidermis and dermis on the lower leg persisting for four weeks or more, but excluding ulcers confined to the foot.

Causes of leg ulceration

Leg ulcers may arise from a number of underlying pathologies. Minor trauma is often the immediate cause of the ulcer, but underlying pathology leads to ulcer development. The most common of these pathologies is venous disease, but a significant number arise from other conditions. It is important to determine the underlying cause because of its implications for the management of the ulcer.

Common causes

Approximately 70 per cent of ulcers are the result of venous disease, usually due to incompetent valves in the deep and perforating veins.

Around 10–15 per cent arise from arterial disease when there is atherosclerotic occlusion of the large vessels or arteritis of the small ones. These changes lead to tissue ischaemia. Diabetes mellitus and rheumatoid arthritis can also alter the smaller distal arteries. In addition, Raynaud's disease affects the arterial circulation.

Approximately 10 per cent of patients will have both venous and arterial disease, and their ulcers will be of mixed aetiology.

Other causes

Around 2–5 per cent of patients develop ulcers from other causes. Although rare, these should be kept in mind. Some of these are listed in Box 8.3.

Box 8.3: Causes of leg ulceration

- Neuropathy – often associated with diabetes mellitus
- Malignancy – basal cell carcinoma, squamous cell carcinoma or melanoma
- Infections – tuberculosis, deep fungal infections, leprosy and syphilis; these are rare in the UK but should be considered, particularly if the patient has been travelling or living in the tropics
- Lymphoedema – usually associated with ulceration following cellulitis only if venous disease is also present (Morison, 1991)
- Metabolic disorders – e.g. Pyoderma gangrenosum
- Blood disorders – e.g. sickle cell disease and thalassaemia
- Self-inflicted ulcers
- Iatrogenic – these can be caused by ill-fitting plaster casts or badly applied bandages being used to treat existing ulcers

---

Assessment

The successful treatment of leg ulcers requires a thorough assessment and diagnosis of the underlying pathology. Assessment should cover the patient's general condition (Box 8.4), the ulcer-related history, clinical investigations and examination of the ulcer itself. Patient assessment and wound assessment have been discussed in some detail above, but an overview and information on issues specific to leg ulcers will be given here.

Ulcer-related history

The assessment of a patient presenting with either a first or a recurrent leg ulcer should include a detailed history of the onset of the problem. A summary of medical histories that may be indicative of venous or arterial disease is shown in Box 8.5.

Box 8.4: Assessment of the patient's general condition

- Age
- Sex
- Family history – there may be a factor(s) predisposing to leg ulcer development
- Occupational history – venous leg ulcers are often associated with occupations involving prolonged standing
- Mobility – reduced mobility contributes to ulcer development and poor healing
- Diet – poor nutritional status may delay healing
- Obesity – may contribute to ulcer development and poor healing
- Smoking habits – may contribute to poor healing and circulatory disease
- General living conditions
- Psychological status – important in determining a patient's participation in care and compliance with treatment

---

Box 8.5: Relevant medical history

A medical history of patients with *venous* disease may include any of the following:

- varicose veins – either treated or untreated;
- deep vein thrombosis;
- phlebitis of the affected leg;
- suspected deep vein thrombosis, e.g. swollen leg following surgery, pregnancy or trauma;
- surgery on the affected leg;
- trauma to the affected leg, such as a fracture;
- history of pulmonary embolism

A medical history suggestive of *arterial* involvement may include:

- hypertension;
- myocardial infarction;
- angina;
- transient ischaemic attacks;
- diabetes mellitus;
- rheumatoid arthritis;
- cerebrovascular accident;
- arterial surgery;
- intermittent claudication;
- peripheral vascular disease

Ulcer-specific history

This should include a history of any previous ulceration, with its duration, the treatments used and any known allergies to dressings. A history of the current episode of ulceration should also be documented.

Clinical investigations

Some routine investigations can aid the diagnosis of the leg ulcer or help in its management. Other investigations, necessary in only a few cases, include weight and tissue biopsy. These are summarized in Table 8.3.

Table 8.3: Clinical investigations

Investigation	Rationale
Blood pressure measurement	To detect hypertension
Urinalysis/BM stick	To detect diabetes
Blood tests	Full blood count and haemoglobin levels to identify anaemia Test for rheumatoid factor
Wound swab	If signs of infection are present, to determine antibiotic sensitivity
Tissue biopsy	If malignancy is suspected
Weight	If patient is obese requiring dietary advice and weight reduction to aid healing

Vascular assessment

The simplest form of vascular assessment is to palpate the foot pulses, both the dorsalis pedis and the posterior tibial. However, the presence of oedema may make these difficult to feel. A more accurate way to ascertain the condition of the arterial circulation is to measure the ankle–brachial pressure index (ABPI) using Doppler ultrasound. This should be done only by a nurse who has received training and has practised under supervision. The brief description given here is not sufficient to enable an untrained nurse to start using this technique. Readers who would like to use this method should contact their local wound care specialist nurse.

Measuring the ABPI

This determines the ratio of the ankle to the brachial systolic pressure with the aid of a battery-operated, hand-held Doppler probe. The patient should lie as flat as possible for at least 10 minutes (Morison and Moffatt 1994) in order to overcome the effects of exercise on the blood pressure. During this time, the patient's history can be taken.

The brachial systolic pressure is recorded for both arms and the higher figure used for calculation (Vowden et al., 1996). An appropriately sized sphygmomanometer cuff is positioned around the arm, and ultrasound gel is placed over the brachial pulse to ensure a good seal between the probe and the skin. The Doppler probe is placed at a slight angle over the brachial pulse until a good signal is heard. The cuff is inflated until the signal disappears and then gradually deflated until the signal returns. This is the brachial systolic pressure.

To take the pressure of the foot pulses, an appropriately sized sphygmomanometer cuff is secured just above the medial malleolus; any open wounds will require covering to prevent contamination either of or from the cuff. The dorsalis pedis, posterior tibial and anterior tibial pulses are located in turn. For each pulse, the cuff is inflated until the signal is lost and then slowly deflated until the signal returns. For maximum accuracy, each pulse should be measured twice. It should be noted that the dorsalis pedis pulse is congenitally absent in up to 12 per cent of people (Barnhorst and Barner, 1968).

To calculate the ABPI, the highest ankle pressure measured is divided by the highest brachial pressure:

$$\text{Ankle brachial pressure index} = \frac{\text{ankle systolic pressure}}{\text{brachial systolic pressure}}$$

The value obtained for the ABPI should normally be greater than 1.0. If the reading obtained is below 1.0, some degree of arterial disease is indicated. An ABPI of 0.90–0.95 indicates minor arterial disease. An ABPI below 0.8 suggests significant arterial disease and compression bandaging is contraindicated. Referral for further vascular assessment is required (Morison and Moffatt, 1994). A ratio of 0.50–0.75 often means that the patient suffers intermittent claudication and below this level ischaemic rest pain, which will require rapid referral to a vascular surgeon.

An ABPI above 1.2 may be pathological. Diabetic patients, for example, may show a falsely high ABPI because of medial calcinosis, vessels being difficult to compress. Compression bandaging should not be applied to diabetic patients except under close medical supervision (Morison and Moffatt, 1994).

If there is any doubt about the ABPI significance of an ABPI, the doctor should be consulted for advice. Anyone who has not been trained to carry out Doppler readings should not attempt this procedure (see accountability, Chapter 1).

Doppler readings should be made when the patient first presents with an episode of ulceration, if the ulcer is deteriorating, if the ulcer is refractory to treatment after three months, and at regular intervals, for example 6-monthly, during treatment.

Examination of the legs and skin

The patient should have both legs thoroughly examined, whether ulcerated or not. Box 8.6 summarizes the clinical signs and symptoms of both venous and arterial disease.

Box 8.6: Signs of venous and arterial disease

Signs of *venous* disease may include:

- varicose veins;
- lipodermatosclerosis (hardening of the dermis and underlying subcutaneous);
- stasis eczema;
- ankle flare (the appearance of many dilated intradermal venules over the medial aspect of the ankle);
- staining of the skin due to breakdown products of haemoglobin from extravasted red blood cells;
- atrophe blanche (areas of white skin with tiny red spots, which are dilated capillary loops)

Signs of *arterial* disease may include:

- cold legs and feet in a warm environment;
- pale or blue feet when raised;
- feet dusky pink when dependant;
- shiny hairless leg;
- gangrenous toes;
- absent foot pulses;
- trophic changes to nails;
- Poor tissue perfusion: if direct pressure is applied to the nail bed, return to normal colour takes longer than 3 seconds

---

Oedema may be present with either venous or arterial disease, but its presence should be noted and other possible causes investigated and eliminated.

Examination of the ulcer

Wound assessment has been discussed in depth above. This section will examine the usual differences between arterial and venous ulcers (Table 8.4).

Table 8.4: Common differences between the appearance of venous and arterial ulcers

	Venous ulcers	Arterial
Site	Often near the medial or lateral malleolus.	Often on the foot or lateral aspect of the leg but may occur anywhere, including the malleolar areas
Depth and shape	Usually shallow with a poorly defined edge	Often deep with a punched out appearance; often irregular shapes or multiple small areas
Pain	The pain of venous ulceration is often associated with oedema, from local infections or cellulitis. Pain can be relieved by support bandages and elevation	Invariably painful. Pain often made worse by elevation or exercise. Patient may report hanging the legs out of bed to relieve pain
Development	Usually slow unless infected	Often rapid

It should be noted that ulcers with a rolled edge or raised ulcer base may be malignant.

Referrals

The vast majority of ulcers will not require further assessment. In some instances, however, further advice and assessment may be required. These include:

- a significantly reduced ABPI – discuss with the general practitioner the need for vascular referral;

- rapid deterioration of the ulcer;
- suspected malignancy;
- newly diagnosed diabetes mellitus;
- signs of contact dermatitis;
- cellulitus;
- ulcers that fail to respond to treatment after a 3-month period.

Some areas may have specialist nurses who may be able to advise in these instances; other areas will be dependent on consultant referral.

Nursing treatment

The aim of treatment is threefold:

- to heal the ulcer;
- to treat the underlying condition;
- to prevent recurrence.

Local ulcer treatment

The choice of dressing will depend upon assessment of the ulcer (see above). In most instances, a simple dressing that is capable of maintaining a moist warm environment conducive to healing should be chosen. Excessive exudate should be absorbed. Dressings should be non-adherent, non-toxic, non-allergenic and non-sensitizing (Morgan, 1987).

Ulcers should be cleansed by irrigation with warm normal saline if necessary. This may not be needed if there is no old dressing material or exudate. The legs may be washed with warm tap water containing an emollient if desired. Infection control issues (see Chapter 3) need to be addressed if using a communal bucket in a general practice. The bucket must be lined with plastic (new for each patient) to prevent cross-infection. Patients may appreciate the opportunity to wash their legs if they are unable to shower or bathe.

The dressing should be changed once a week unless there is excessive exudate, discomfort or bandage slippage (NHSE, 1995). However, the treatment regime should be determined in conjunction with the patient, and there will be instances when more frequent changes are necessary (see patient autonomy, Chapter 1).

Contact sensitivity to treatment may occur at any time. Patients with reactions to unknown sensitizers should be referred to a dermatologist for patch testing. In cases of sensitivity, remove the known or potential allergen, apply a simple non-adherent dressing, and elevate and rest the limb. Liaise with the general practitioner to prescribe a steroid ointment (as cream may contain sensitizers). Apply the ointment for 2–4 days. Reduce the amount of steroid used over the following 3–4 days, and replace the steroid with white soft paraffin emollient.

Assess the pain level when there is pain at the wound site. Consider whether the dressing may be causing pain by adherence, and, if necessary, change to a less adherent product. Compression therapy, exercise and elevation may relieve the pain of patients who have venous ulceration. Analgesia should be tailored to meet individual patient requirements. In extreme cases, opiate analgesia may be required.

All patients should be offered accessible and appropriate information on their leg ulcer disease. This should include the rationale for treatment, self-help strategies, the services available to them, dietary advice and lifestyle advice. Many manufacturing companies produce comprehensive patient booklets that can be obtained from representatives. Consider using your own educational and health promotion skills.

Treating the underlying condition

This is the most important part of leg ulcer treatment. Unless the underlying condition is treated, the ulcer is unlikely to respond to treatment.

Venous ulceration

If arterial involvement has been excluded, the underlying venous disorder should be treated with compression bandaging, exercise and elevation.

Exercise

Walking will exercise the calf muscle and work the muscle pump, increasing venous return. Regular flexion and extension exercises are beneficial in working the calf muscle pump for patients with limited mobility. Exercise aids, such as the C'aire Cush, may also be beneficial. These can be bought at some pharmacies.

Elevation

Patients should be encouraged to elevate their legs above hip height when sitting to facilitate venous return.

Compression

Graduated compression will assist venous return and improve muscle pump function. The suggested level of compression is between 20 and 40 mmHg at the ankle, and 50 per cent of that value at the knee (Kendrick et al., 1994). A compression bandage should be anchored at the base of the toes, exert maximum compression at the ankle and finish at the knee.

Manufacturers' instructions for application should be followed. Bandages that are incorrectly applied are at best uncomfortable and useless, and at worst dangerous. Patients with an ABPI of less than 0.8 must not have compression therapy.

Single layer compression, such as Surepress (Contavec) or Tensopress (Smith & Nephew), should be applied to manufacturers' instructions. Padding may be required under the bandaging to protect the leg, particularly over bony prominences. Patients with an ankle circumference of less than 18 cm are not suitable for compression bandaging unless sufficient padding is applied to build up the ankle size.

Multilayer compression systems should provide adequate padding, adequate compression and sustained compression for at least a week. In most instances, a weekly dressing change is recommended. Only accepted systems should be used. These may come in kit form such as Profore, or bandages may be purchased separately. All patients should have their ankle circumference measured to ensure that the appropriate bandage regime is selected. Manufacturers' instructions for application should be adhered to, and practitioners must be appropriately trained in the application of multilayer bandaging.

Arterial and mixed-aetiology ulceration

Unless advised to the contrary, for example by a vascular surgeon, mixed-aetiology ulcers should be treated as arterial. Compression must not be used on ulcers with a substantial arterial component. Any bandages used should be light retention bandages only.

Mild exercise and ankle exercise should be encouraged, particularly if the patient is immobile. Pain control may be achieved by rest, analgesia and a suitable dressing, for example hydrocolloid or hydrogel.

Patients with arterial disease, particularly those with an ABPI below 0.75, should be considered for a surgical opinion.

Diabetic and rheumatoid ulceration

These ulcers are often difficult to manage. There is often substantial arterial involvement arising from the peripheral vascular changes associated with these diseases.

Rheumatoid ulceration may show no signs of circulatory disorders, and diabetic ulceration may be complicated by peripheral neuropathy. If either of these conditions is suspected but undiagnosed, a medical opinion should be sought. Both of these groups of ulcer should be treated as arterial, with rest, pain control, monitoring of the associated disease and early consultant referral.

Summary

Individual healing rates will vary whatever the underlying condition, but any ulcer not responding to treatment in 4–8 weeks should be reassessed. Treatment may need to be changed, or the patient may require further investigations or referral to either a consultant or a specialist nurse.

Advice to prevent recurrence is essential as approximately 75 per cent of patients will suffer from this, and it can be reduced if appropriate advice is given.

Patients should be advised to report any new leg damage as soon as possible so that treatment can begin. Patients with venous disease require compression therapy for life. When healing is complete, they should be measured for suitable hosiery. Compliance is more likely with below-knee stockings, which are relatively easy to put on. Although class 3 stockings (delivering a compression of 25–35 mmHg) are desirable, a patient with dexterity problems may be encouraged to comply by moving down to class 2 (a compression of 18–24 mmHg). Patients should be encouraged to continue with exercise, and advice on diet, lifestyle and smoking habits should be reinforced. The legs will need to be protected against trauma damage, and the underlying disease will be monitored.

Key points:

1. Practice nurses have an important role to play in wound management in the primary care setting.
2. It is important to keep up to date with new treatment methods but, at the same time, to acknowledge any limitations in wound management and to refer the patient for specialist advice if necessary.
3. The patients' role in the management of their wounds should be appreciated, and they should be involved in the planning of their care and future management.

4. All wounds are unique and will respond differently to treatment. This chapter provides guidelines to optimize wound healing, but the experience of working with many wounds, and trying to achieve rapid healing, will be the greatest guides.

References

Angeras MH, Brandberg A, Falk A, Seeman T (1991) Comparison between sterile saline and tap water for the cleansing of acute traumatic soft tissue wounds. European Journal of Surgery 158(33): 347–50.

Barnhorst DA, Barner HB (1968) Prevalence of congenitally absent foot pulses. New England Journal of Medicine 278: 264–5.

Cherry GW, Ryan TJ (1985) Enhanced wound angiogenesis with a new hydrocolloid dressing. In Ryan TJ (Ed.) An environment for healing. The role of occlusion. International Congress and Symposium. Series No. 88. London: Royal Society of Medicine.

Chrintz H (1989) Need for surgical wound dressings. British Journal of Surgery 76: 204–5.

Cooper R, Lawrence JC (1996) The isolation and identification of bacteria from wounds. Journal of Wound Care 5(7): 335–40.

Cutting KF, Harding KG (1994) Criteria for identifying wound infection. Journal of Wound Care 3(4): 198–201.

David J (1986) Wound Management. A Comprehensive Guide to Dressing and Healing. London: Martin Dunitz.

Dealey C (1994) The Care of Wounds: A Guide for Nurses. Oxford: Blackwell Scientific Publications.

Draper J (1985) Making the dressing fit the wound. Nursing Times 81(4): 32–5.

Dyson M, Young S, Pendle C (1988) Comparison of the effects of moist and dry conditions on dermal repair. Journal of Investigative Dermatology 91(5): 435–49.

Hutchinson JJ, Lawrence JC (1991) Wound infection under occlusive dressings. Journal of Hospital Infection 17: 83–4.

Kendrick M, Lucker K, Cullum N, Roe B (1994) Clinical Information Pack No. 1: The Management of Leg Ulcers in the Community. Liverpool: University of Liverpool.

Lawrence JC (1997) Wound irrigation. Journal of Wound Care 6(1): 23–6.

Lock PM (1980) The effect of temperature on mitotic activity at the edge of experimental wounds. In Lundgren A, Soner AB (Eds) Symposia on Wound Healing: Plastic, Surgical and Dermatologic Aspects. Sweden: Molndal.

Miller M (1995) Wound care for minor injuries. Primary Health Care 5(10): 23–6.

Miller M, Dyson M (1996) The Principles of Wound Care. London: Macmillan.

Morgan D (1987) Formulary of Wound Management Products. Cardiff: Whitchurch Hospital.

Morgan D (1994) Formulary of Wound Management Products, 6th Edn. Haslemere: Euromed Communications.

Morison M (1991) A Colour Guide to the Assessment and Management of Leg Ulcers. London: Wolfe Publishing.

Morison M (1992) A Colour Guide to the Management of Wounds. London: Wolfe Publishing.

Morison M, Moffatt C (1994) A Colour Guide to the Assessment and Management of Leg Ulcers, 2nd Edn. London: CV Mosby.

Myers JA (1982) Wound healing and the use of a modern surgical dressing. Pharmaceutical Journal 229(6186): 103–4.

National Health Service Executive (1995) Consensus Strategy For Management of Leg Ulcers. London: NHSE.

Newman V, Allwood M, Oakes R (1989) The use of metronidazole gel to control the smell of malodorous lesions. Palliative Medicine 3(4): 303–5.

Nursing Times (1994) Wound care. Knowledge for practice. Professional Development Series. Nursing Times 90: 49.

Plewa M (1990) Altered host response and special infections in the elderly. Emergency Medicine Clinics of North America 8(2): 193–206.

Reid J, Morison M (1994) Towards a consensus classification of pressure sores. Journal of Wound Care 3(3): 293–4.

Silver IA (1985) Oxygen and tissue repair. In Ryan TJ (Ed.) An Environment for Healing: The Role of Occlusion. International Congress and Symposium. Series No. 88. London: Royal Society of Medicine.

Thomas S (1990) Wound Management and Dressings. London: Pharmaceutical Press.

Thompson PD, Smith DJ (1994) What is infection? American Journal of Surgery 67a (supplement): 75–115.

Vowden KR, Goulding V, Vowden P (1996) Hand-held Doppler assessment for peripheral arterial disease. Journal of Wound Care 5(3): 125–8.

Winter G (1962) Formation of the scab and the rate of epithelialization of superficial wounds in the skin of the young domestic pig. Nature 193: 293–4.

Chapter 9
The future for practice nursing

Marilyn Edwards

The future for practice nurses who wish to develop and expand their role is challenging. This chapter offers an insight into the development of practice nursing over the past 30 years. The role of the practice nurse has been enhanced through recent educational opportunities, which enable nurses to develop their skills to meet the needs of their practice population. Social policy has not been included in this book because of its complexity; nurses must be prepared to deliver quality care despite political vagaries and social policy.

Practice nursing has developed from a task-orientation role within a treatment room to professional nursing with specialist skills and knowledge. Practice nurses' development has in the past suffered because of the lack of management structure, the absence of support from health authorities, and a limited availability of appropriately qualified practice nurse lecturers or assessors. Many nurses work in isolation and have little peer support.

The practice nurse today is more likely be an autonomous practitioner than a handmaiden to the doctor. Universities and schools of nursing are constantly developing the education and training requirements of nurses to meet this changing and challenging role. This final chapter outlines the rise of practice nursing and examines some of the more recent developments in the changing role of the practice nurse.

The practice nurse

Practice nurses are generally level 1 nurses, employed by general practitioners to perform clinical and preventive health care procedures in the surgery.

According to Rashid et al. (1996), a practice nurse works with a general practitioner and is responsible for implementing prescribed programmes of care under the supervision of the general practitioner. A modern definition may read 'a practice nurse works with a general practitioner to devise and implement programmes of health care for a defined population'.

The position of practice nurse has evolved since the early 1970s. Historically, district nurses saw patients in general practitioner premises as well as in their own homes, but the time available proved insufficient for patient needs. General practitioners began to employ their own nurses, enabling the general practitioners to work more effectively and efficiently, and making it possible for practices to offer an increased range of services. A 70 per cent subsidy, introduced for salary reimbursement in the mid-1960s, encouraged general practitioners to employ a nurse in the practice to whom the doctor could delegate some of the clinical work.

The number of practice nurses has increased steadily since 1977, although figures vary between authors (Table 9.1). The rapid expansion in number since 1990 is a consequence of changes in the contractual requirements of general practice, which had an emphasis on health promotion.

Nurses enter general practice from backgrounds ranging from extensive community experience (health visiting, district nursing, school nursing or midwifery) to experience only in their general training. There is no standard agreement on either the qualifications necessary for the job or the objectives for professional development: individual nurses and their employers decide their own terms.

A national census of practice nurses reported that 99.9 per cent of practice nurses are women and 97 per cent are white (Atkin et al., 1993). This raises concerns about sexual and ethnic equality and discrimination within the profession. It might be pertinent to determine whether or not these minorities apply for practice nurse posts. If not, what are the reasons for their lack of interest? Action might

Table 9.1: Growth of practice nursing

Year	Approx no. of practice nurses	Reference
1977	1 500	Stilwell (1991)
1986	4 000	Greenfield et al. (1987)
1990	8 155	Ross et al. (1994)
1993	16 000	Atkin et al. (1993)

then be taken to redress this inequality in areas where it would have a positive impact on the health care provided by the practice.

The poorly defined role of the practice nurse, and the overlap of community nurse roles, was highlighted in the census. Practice nurses and district nurses both undertook home visits, whilst practice nurses and health visitors had an educational/preventive role. District nurses and health visitors can either feel threatened by, or welcome, the flexible role of the practice nurse. Health visitors are recognized as health educators, although many practice nurses undertake this role without appropriate training. This is addressed in current higher education courses and through local health education authority initiatives, although not all nurses are able to take advantage of such training opportunities.

A study in 1987 examining the working practices of 300 practice nurses revealed enormous variations in patterns of work (Greenfield et al., 1987). The authors concluded that the majority of nurses felt that their role could be extended, although some nurses wished to shed traditional nursing tasks, such as ear syringing, giving injections and removing sutures. It was not indicated who should do these tasks. The study results suggest that some nurses would be happy moving away from the traditional caring role of nursing.

Ross et al. (1994) reported in their study of workload and training needs that some nurses were carrying out tasks for which they were overqualified, such as cleaning, and others were engaged in patient care activities for which they had no formal training. The ability to delegate safely, and issues of professional accountability, are essential ingredients of professional nursing.

Practice nurses rarely manage other practice nurses, although general practitioners have identified a clear role for a senior nurse to co-ordinate nursing resources (Atkin and Lunt, 1995).

The lack of a managerial structure allowing practice nurses a certain degree of autonomy is reflected in individual nursing practice. Nurses who work in a team without an identified manager may encounter friction within the team, while nurses who work in isolation may view their employer as their manager. Nurses who work within an integrated nursing team may currently be managed by a health visitor or district nurse. Practice nurses may wish to discuss realistic management structures with their employers; practice nurse status will increase when a practice nurse is appointed team leader over other disciplines.

Accountability

The General Medical Council's guidance 'Good Medical Practice' allows doctors to delegate medical care to nurses if they are sure that the nurses are competent to undertake the work, the doctor remaining responsible for managing the patient's care (GMC, 1995).

Although the doctor takes vicarious liability for the nurse's actions, the nurse is professionally accountable for her own actions (UKCC, 1992a). The fact remains that some nurses still appear to undertake tasks for which they are not appropriately trained. This may be a result of pressure on general practitioners to delegate down, a fear of job losses in areas of low employment and/or a poor appreciation of individual accountability and liability. Patient care can be compromised by potentially incompetent care. The nurse also places herself at risk of disciplinary action (see Chapter 1).

Community health care nursing

Community health care nurses have been defined as 'nurses who have completed a specific post-registration preparation in order to provide a skilled nursing service to the community' (UKCC, 1991). Practice nurses were not included in the list of existing practitioners in 1991, although the guidelines were expanded in 1993.

Automatic recognition as a community health care nurse was awarded to nurses who:

- had already completed an appropriate recordable or registerable post-registration community nursing course of no less than six months in length; and
- had at least two years registered practice in the appropriate area. (UKCC, 1993)

The 'Report on Proposals for the Future of Community Education and Practice' (UKCC, 1991) aimed to develop cohesive, proactive community health care nurses able to determine nursing policies relevant and responsive to the health needs of the population.

Current community health degrees combine an academic degree with a recordable practice nurse qualification. The graduate is then a community health care nurse. Many practice nurses, who are not community health care nurses by definition, are already undertaking some of the tasks listed in the report, summarized in Box 9.1.

Box 9.1: Skills of the community health care nurse (UKCC, 1991, para. 19)

The community health care nurse is trained to:

- use a proactive approach to health by searching for, and identifying, evolving health care needs and situations hazardous to health;
- stimulate an awareness of health needs to promote positive and healthy lifestyles;
- empower people to take appropriate action to influence health policies;
- provide leadership, management and teaching skills to ensure quality and continuity of care;
- provide health data through health profiles;
- undertake forms of audit, review and appropriate quality assurance activities

---

Training

An English National Board (ENB) review of the education and training of practice nurses recommended the provision of education at different levels, including 'employment-led' induction programmes and 'education-led' advanced courses (ENB, 1990). This addressed the haphazard opportunities for training that had previously existed.

Study days and updates are provided on an *ad hoc* basis by district health authorities (DHA), which superseded family health service authorities (FHSAs), but they do not necessarily meet the needs of individual nurses. Although these events are usually funded by the employer and/or the DHA, a lack of flexibility may prevent more than one nurse from a practice attending, particularly when no alternative dates or venues are available. Study days commissioned by the Health Authorities are often expensive but are usually more flexible.

Post-registration education and practice (PREP) has made it compulsory for nurses constantly to advance their practice through learning, but certificated learning experience is not required.

In-house training is particularly valuable when topics include specific areas of disease processes and patient management. Nurses should not feel uncomfortable asking their employers for such training.

A variety of courses are now available via academic centres and open learning. These include academic degrees, diplomas and certificates covering asthma, cervical cytology, diabetes and counselling. However, funding for, and the time available to attend, these courses will vary between general practices. Nurses should ensure that study leave is incorporated into their contract of employment.

Practice nurses must be competent to deliver the care required in general practice. The original registerable qualification does not meet this criterion. Nurses who enter practice nursing via the Project 2000 nurse training will already be grounded in health and health promotion theory. Current post-registration courses place an emphasis on health and health promotion, which are essential components of general practice work.

Practice nurses appear to underestimate their future training needs according to Atkin et al. (1993), who question whether practice nurses are adequately trained to undertake health promotion (traditionally a health visitor role).

Practice nurses surveyed by Atkin and Lunt in a later study (1995) expressed their concern about the need for continuing education and training to develop their role, although a small proportion of nurses had not received any training in the previous year. General practitioners largely supported the idea of continuing training for nurses but did not actively encourage nurses to attend courses.

In theory, as nurses become more highly skilled, their status will be reflected in higher grading. The increased cost to the practice may be offset through skill mix, some team members having less training and proportionately lower pay grades. However, this scenario is not appropriate for nurses who work in isolation. Grading and pay should ideally reflect education and expertise rather than merely what the employing doctor is prepared to pay.

Nurse practitioners

Currently, any nurse is free to use the title of 'nurse practitioner', although the UKCC states in the final report on PREP that it does not recognize this term as all nurses are practitioners in their own right (UKCC, 1993).

Castledine (1995) defines a nurse practitioner as 'A registered nurse who has been specially prepared to carry out and integrate a more medical model of care into his/her nursing practice, with the purpose of improving health assessment, management and delivery of services at the first level of access.'

Development of the nurse practitioner

The nurse practitioner was introduced in the USA during the late 1960s in response to a shortage of physicians and was very much a doctor-substitute role. Barbara Stilwell pioneered the role in the UK in the 1970s in the firm belief that the nurse practitioner would advance the contribution of nursing within primary health care. The nurse practitioner was initially involved in five key areas of work (Box 9.2).

Box 9.2 The nurse practitioner (Stilwell, 1984)

- Acts as an alternative consultant for the patient
- Detects serious disease by physical examination
- Manages minor and chronic ailments and injuries
- Provides health education
- Counsels

The role of the nurse practitioner in the UK developed from government concerns about cost-effectiveness in health care, highlighted by the Cumberlege Report (DoH, 1986). A study undertaken in Birmingham in the early 1980s concluded that, when given a choice between a nurse practitioner and a medical practitioner, most patients chose a consultation with the nurse practitioner appropriately (Stilwell et al., 1987). The nurse practitioner managed the presenting problem without further referral for investigation, prescription or other medical advice. There were no reported cases of serious illness going unnoticed.

Stilwell (1988) cites evidence that nurse practitioners provide care that is equivalent to, and sometimes more effective than, that of physicians, particularly in the care of patients with chronic disease. Although the nurse is cheaper to employ than a doctor, consultations are often longer, so nurses must not be seen as a cheap alternative to physicians. The emphasis on health promotion and preventive medicine has made it difficult to evaluate the true costs of health care.

The role of the nurse practitioner has been recognized as being a means of improving primary health care, particularly with relation to client choice, satisfaction and the inequalities that exist in service provision and usage (Whitehead, 1988). Nurse practitioners have been instrumental in reducing some of the inequalities in health both in less developed countries and among disadvantaged groups in the UK, demonstrated by the frequent reports in nursing journals on health care for the homeless.

The role of nurse practitioner may vary between practitioners but is likely to encompass a caring rather than a medical curing role (Box 9.3). Many practice nurses will be undertaking this role even though they may not be calling themselves nurse practitioners.

Box 9.3: Competencies of the nurse practitioner

- Offering direct access to primary health care
- Assessing the health of clients with undifferentiated and undiagnosed conditions by utilizing verbal and physical examination techniques
- Differentiating between abnormal and normal findings with reference to disease and illness states
- Initiating treatment and care falling within his or her range of knowledge and skills
- Evaluating care and treatment, and discharging clients from the primary health care system as appropriate
- Making autonomous decisions and exercising professional accountability
- Providing instruction and counselling to clients, particularly in relation to health promotion and maintenance
- Referring clients to physicians and other agencies where necessary

---

The practice nurse working as a nurse practitioner could offer an alternative to general practitioner consultation, although it may be argued that the role falls within a medical remit. General practitioners vary in their acceptance of nurses in this role; innovative general practitioners actively encourage nurse practitioner education.

The authors of one study of 620 nurses working in general practice suggest that, whilst the majority of nurses perform a wide range of delegated tasks, nearly half have extended their role towards independent practice (Ross et al., 1994).

Marsh and Dawes (1995) have demonstrated that appropriately trained nurses are competent to diagnose and manage minor illnesses in general practice. Half of the patients in their study required only advice on self-care, with or without a recommendation for over-the-counter drugs. It is probable that many experienced practice nurses are currently undertaking this role unofficially.

The results of the South Thames Regional Health Authority experience suggest that nurse practitioners can improve the quality of and choice within primary care by offering patients a choice of professional and consultation style (Fawcett Henesy and West, 1995). Although most of the nurse practitioners' consultations were longer than those of general practitioners, consultation time reduced as nurse practitioners' confidence developed. There is a clear role for both doctors and nurses, with complementary skills, when roles and responsibilities are clearly defined.

The Royal College of Nursing (RCN) has clarified some of the issues surrounding the title and role of the nurse practitioner and believes that only those nurses who have completed a course of specific education for the role should use the title (RCN, 1997a). The criteria for identifying a nurse practitioner are listed in Box 9.4.

Box 9.4: Criteria for identifying a trained nurse practitioner (RCN, 1997a)

- Manages his or her own caseload
- Has undertaken a specific course of study to at least first degree level
- Makes professionally autonomous decisions
- Assesses the health care needs of previously undiagnosed patients
- Screens patients/clients for disease risk factors and early signs of disease
- Negotiates a health care plan with the patient/client
- Counsels and offers health education
- Refers to other health care providers

Nurse practitioners may be cheaper to employ, but they have longer consultations than doctors, so the cost effectiveness of this role in practice is difficult to assess.

The expertise of the primary care nurse practitioner is parallel to that of a general practitioner operating as a 'specialist generalist' (RCN, 1997a). Nurse practitioners offer an alternative source of care complementary to that of the general practitioner. They should not be treated as doctor substitutes.

Nurse prescribing

Nurse prescribing is an acknowledgment and endorsement of the current contribution of nurses to patient care and a recognition of the need to supply items necessary for effective nursing treatment (Andrews, 1994).

The concept of nurse prescribing evolved from the report 'Neighbourhood Nursing – a Focus for Care' (DoH, 1986), which stated: 'The DHSS should agree a limited list of items and simple agents which may be prescribed by nurses as part of a nursing care programme.'

An advisory group on nurse prescribing led to the Crown Report (DoH, 1989), which defined three areas in which nurses would be able to prescribe (Box 9.5). Eight demonstration sites were chosen to pilot nurse prescribing from a limited formulary, referred to as the Nurses Formulary. Only nurses with a district nurse or health visitor qualification were eligible in September 1994 to undertake the necessary training to enable them to be entered on the UKCC register; they included practice nurses with a health visitor or district nurse qualification.

Box 9.5: Areas in which it was proposed by the Crown Report that nurses would be able to prescribe

- The initial prescribing from a limited list of items – the Nurses Formulary
- Supplying medicines within group protocols, e.g. immunizations
- Adjusting the timing and dosage of medication prescribed by a medical practitioner within clearly defined protocols

---

The benefit of nurse prescribing to patients and clients has been acknowledged by Winstanley (1996) and the Department of Health (DOH; 1989), and is summarized in Box 9.6. [box 9.6 here]

Box 9.6: Benefits of nurse prescribing for the practice nurse

- A service that is more appropriate and responsive to patient needs
- A better, faster and more cost-effective treatment of minor but potentially serious and therefore costly conditions
- A more appropriate use of nurses' extensive professional skills
- Increased nurse autonomy and satisfaction
- An increased awareness of prescribing costs
- An increased awareness of over-the-counter products
- A saving on general practitioner appointment time
- An improved working relationship with medical colleagues

The government White Paper 'Primary Care: Delivering the Future' (DoH, 1996a) extended nurse prescribing to approximately 500 nurses from 1500 practices. As from April 1998, nurse prescribing was to be further extended to all qualified district nurses and health visitors in England, allowing them to prescribe drugs for chronic illnesses that had already been diagnosed by a doctor. It is hoped that the next step will be the extension of nurse prescribing to include practice nurses.

If the primary role of the nurse is to enable independence and interdependence (Andrews, 1994), prescribing must be seen within this context. When prescribing, supplying or altering the timing or dosage of an item, nurses have the opportunity to engage actively in health teaching and question whether any prescription is required at all. Although many items in the Nurses Formulary are readily available over the counter, members of the public expect infinitely more knowledge and expertise from a nurse who prescribes than when choosing a product for themselves.

The RCN (1995) advocates extending prescribing rights to all community health care nurses (Box 9.7).

> **Box 9.7: Extending prescribing rights (RCN, 1995)**
>
> - The inclusion of practice nurses and those working in minor injury clinics
> - Expanding the Nurses Formulary to include any item that a community nurse would use in the delivery of nursing care, including oral contraceptives
> - A comprehensive education programme for all community nurses who wished to prescribe
> - The establishment of a standing nurse formulary committee to receive requests from the profession for additional formulary items
> - The adoption of a nationally accepted system through which nurses could provide non-nurse formulary items with the agreement of a medical practitioner

Group protocols

Jones and Gough (1997) explain the development and legality of group protocols, which were identifed as essential practice for improving patient care by the Crown Report (DoH, 1989). No legislation has been passed to legalize the use of protocols and, despite efforts by the professional bodies, the DoH has not yet clarified the situation.

Group protocols have been used under Section 58(2)(a) and (b) of the Medicines Act 1968, which states that prescription-only medicines can be administered against a direction from a doctor. Written protocols are commonly used in child immunization programmes, travel clinics and nurse-led family planning clinics. These must be signed by a medical practitioner to be a 'directive'. Guidelines for the administration of medicines were issued by the UKCC in 1992 (UKCC 1992b).

The benefits of using a group protocol have been reported by family planning nurses in the Mersey region, although some nurses were hesitant to accept their new autonomous and accountable role (Thomson, 1996). There appears to be a dearth of literature about the use of group protocols in general practice. This is an area that might merit research by an interested practice nurse.

A group protocol will usually:

- list the criteria against which certain medicines can be supplied or administered to individuals in specific circumstances;
- name those nurses who are competent to undertake this activity;
- be signed by the doctor;
- be used instead of individual prescriptions.

Although nurse prescribing is limited to the Nurses Formulary, it is a legal requirement for nurse practitioners to have prescriptions for other treatments countersigned by a doctor. This reduces the autonomy of the nurse practitioner and wastes both professional and patient time. The profession awaits full prescribing rights for nurse practitioners. Not all nurses will wish to prescribe, but for those who do, appropriate training and support must be available.

Nurses may encounter opposition from some doctors who feel threatened by the expanding role of the nurse. Doctors should perhaps be grateful that nurses are willing to train and be accountable for this enhanced role, which reduces role overlap and improves efficiency in health care service delivery.

Nurses must be fully aware of, and prepared for, the implications of nurse prescribing in terms of autonomy, responsibility and authority, which are based on individual assessment and care requirements. It is essential for individual nurses to explore the extent of professional indemnity insurance.

Specialist practice

The UKCC has recognized that general practice nursing encompasses a wide range of nursing skills and is an area that requires a specialist qualification (UKCC, 1994a).

The Registrar's letter (UKCC, 1994b) laid out the standards required for post-registration education leading to the qualification of specialist practitioner. This will enable practitioners to exercise higher levels of judgement and discretion in clinical care (Box 9.8). Patients and clients should have access to specialist care wherever nursing care is given, although not all practitioners need to become specialists.

Box 9.8: Specialist practitioners

Specialist practitioners are expected to:
- demonstrate higher levels of clinical decision-making;
- monitor and improve standards of care through the supervision of practice;
- undertake clinical audit;
- provide skilled professional leadership;
- develop practice through research;
- teach and support professional colleagues

Qualification of specialist practitioner

The UKCC and National Boards published a statement in June 1996 that aimed to clarify the position with respect to the use of the title 'specialist practitioner' (UKCC, 1996).

A specialist qualification, which will be recorded on the UKCC register, can be obtained by undertaking one of the new programmes approved by a National Board to meet the UKCC's standards, which is no less than first degree level.

Institutions approved for these programmes have assessment of prior learning (APL) mechanisms in place to ensure that maximum credit is offered for appropriate prior learning and learning from experience (APEL).

Transitional arrangements for the title 'specialist practitioner'

Until 31 October 1998, transitional arrangements were made for nurses wishing to obtain the specialist practitioner qualification.

A practice nurse may use the title 'specialist practitioner' if he or she has obtained a post-registration, recordable practice nurse qualification that lasted at least four months, and is also deemed competent under the terms of 'The Scope of Professional Practice' (UKCC, 1992a) and 'Code of Professional Conduct' (UKCC, 1992c). The UKCC will record qualifications obtained from a recognized course commenced on or before 31 October 1998.

Nurses who have had at least five years experience in practice nursing, but who have not obtained a post-registration practice nurse qualification, can apply to nursing institutes for APEL. A good portfolio that demonstrates reflective practice may also be credited. A fee is payable for this service.

It may be argued that the critical and analytical skills of these practitioners do not compare favourably with the skills of those who have undertaken formal development routes, although their clinical skills may be greater. The validity of the title may be questioned when practitioners have not followed the same route of assessment and experience.

In 1997, the UKCC appointed a steering group to define and clarify specialist practice in an attempt to tackle the confusion that surrounded the issue of specialist nurses, especially the role of the nurse practitioner.

Advanced practice

Advanced nursing practice is:

> concerned with adjusting the boundaries for the development of future practice, pioneering and developing new roles responsive to changing needs and with advancing clinical practice, research and education to enrich professional practice as a whole. (UKCC, 1994a)

The UKCC expected nurses to undertake a Master's degree if they wished to work in advanced nursing practice, which would contribute to health policy and management, determine health need and develop these new roles to meet changing practice.

Elcock (1996) has explored the issue of 'consultant nurse' as an appropriate title for the 'advanced nurse practitioner' but concluded that the title is élitist and inappropriate. Although it is stated that consultees can take or leave a consultant's advice, it can be argued that all patients should have the right to accept or decline health care advice or treatment, which weakens the argument against consultancy.

In 1997 the UKCC agreed unanimously that no definition or criteria should be set against which to measure advanced practice, as nurses should be constantly advancing their practice. Most nurse practitioner graduates fulfil the requirements of specialist rather than advanced practice (UKCC, 1997).

Skill mix

Smith (1993) suggests that the term 'grade mix' is more appropriate than 'skill mix' to describe a team where members have mixed skills and expertise. Skill mix has been used in secondary care since the word 'delegation' entered nursing, but Rashid et al. (1996) found little research relating to skill mix in primary care.

Skill can be defined in terms of a number of variables, such as experience, knowledge or qualifications (Richardson and Maynard, 1995).

Skill mix can be applied throughout general practice as the continuing shift from secondary to primary care has led to a corresponding increase in community nurse and medical workload. General practitioners rely on skill mix to deliver quality primary care as fewer doctors enter general practice, and nurses are expected to fill the gap.

The literature suggests that between 30 per cent and 70 per cent of tasks performed by doctors could be carried out by nurses, although studies into the cost-effectiveness of doctor–nurse substitution have not been properly evaluated (Richardson and Maynard, 1995).

A study on the nurse-led management of minor illness in a general practitioner surgery concluded that the nurse appeared able to deal with almost all the patients' presenting problems, offering an extension of patient choice (Rees and Kinnersley, 1996). However, the authors expressed concern that nurses might take on too many responsibilities, which would be detrimental to the health care they offered.

Nursing roles in general practice must develop to meet the needs of the practice within an increasingly limited budget. Future development may include introducing health care assistants to undertake delegated tasks under the training and supervision of practice nurses (Box 9.9).

Box 9.9: Recommendations for health care assistants (HCAs) (RCN, 1997b)

- HCAs should have been trained to NVQ level 3
- Patients must be aware of the difference between a nurse and an HCA
- Delegated tasks should be appropriate and take account of individual abilities
- Procedures needing nursing skills and clinical judgement should not be delegated to an HCA
- Results of clinical measurements should be reported to a nurse or doctor for a decision on a course of action
- A system will be in place to ensure that concerns about practice standards can be reported and action taken

---

Wiltshire FHSA introduced a clinical nurse assistant post as a trial in one fundholding general practice in 1993 (Fairfield, 1996). Following NVQ level 3 training, the clinical nurse assistant was able to undertake treatment room tasks previously undertaken by a G grade nurse or member of the reception staff. The practice subsequently reduced the number of G grade hours. The cost implications of the training and assessment of a candidate in an area with few NVQ assessors include those of the trainee requiring a trainer, mentor and assessor.

The benefits of employing a clinical nurse assistant in general practice will depend upon each nurse's perception. Will the clinical nurse assistant role devalue the practice nurse role, or will it enable the practice nurse to use his or her skills more effectively? There is no doubt that many practice nurses are overqualified for some of the tasks they undertake. Less skilled nurses should be used to assist, rather than replace, qualified nurses.

Cooper (1997) describes how the introduction of a clinical assistant within her general practice has led to a flexible practice team. The assistant receives ongoing training that allows her to develop skills from clerical support to clinical tasks. Practices may already have unoffical health care assistants by virtue of their reception/clerical staff undertaking many of the tasks for which Cooper's assistant was employed.

An appropriately trained clinical nurse assistant can complement the practice nurse to offer a cost-effective service to patients. This will enhance the job satisfaction of both roles. The RCN views skill mix as a more appropriate use of nursing skills rather than a cost-cutting exercise (RCN, 1997b).

Figure 9.1 offers a hypothetical skill and grade mix that reflects the expertise of the practitioner. This would not be feasible where only one or two nurses were employed. Combinations of expertise should reflect the needs of the practice.

Atkin and Lunt (1995) reported that although a division of labour (skill mix) was found in practices employing more than one nurse, this did not necessarily include grade mix. Fundholding practices appeared to have a clearer delineation of nurses' roles.

It could be argued that clinical judgement is a vital component of all nursing interventions, from urinalysis and weight checks to hypertension monitoring. Health care assistants will not have the assessment skills that nurses have attained through years of experience. If they are expected to undertake these tasks, should they therefore consider nurse training?

Practice nurse – G/H grade	team leader
Practice nurse – F/G grade	skilled practitioner
Practice nurse – E grade	treatment room nurse
HCA – B/C grade	trained to meet practice needs and assist other grades

Figure 9.1: A hypothetical grade mix which reflects skill or expertise.

Clinical supervision

Clinical supervision is an interactive process between providers of health care, which enables the development of professional knowledge and skills (Butterworth and Faugier, 1993). The aim of clinical supervision is to encourage professional development and support for nursing staff in order to ensure a high standard of clinical and managerial practice.

Clinical supervision for practice nurses has not developed in the same way as for other nursing hierarchies, partly because of the poorly defined role of practice nurses, who have no requirement to demonstrate their competence formally. Although some general practitioners undertake an 'educative' aspect of supervision, delivered through on-the-job training, 'supportive' supervision is rare.

The rise in practice nurse numbers led to the old FHSAs appointing nurse advisers to support practice nurses professionally, although input to individual nurses inevitably varies between regions, advisers and nurses. The future role and security of the facilitator/adviser is uncertain.

The need for clinical supervision for practice nurses has been recognized and addressed in North Staffordshire, where the value of supervision by an experienced practice nurse was demonstrated through a consensus workshop (Cook and Leech, 1996). It was recommended that a group of 6–10 nurses met monthly with a supervisor to discuss a range of topics and offer peer group support.

This concept could be incorporated into practice nurse groups, especially where nurses work in isolation. Reflection on past experiences through discussion offers nurses the opportunity to increase their self-awareness and meet individual professional needs, leading in turn to a higher quality of patient care. Clinical supervision offers nurses the opportunity to self-evaluate critically all aspects of their clinical experiences, including their successes and errors.

Nurses may be more comfortable using the term 'clinical support' in place of 'clinical supervision'. 'Support' more accurately describes the concept, whilst 'supervision' conjures up observation and assessment.

Partnerships

Nurses and doctors often have conflicting views of partnership, which may relate to the doctor's previous dominant role over the nurse-handmaiden. Partnerships can differ, from total equality or profit-sharing only, to part-partnerships. There has been increasing interest in equal partnerships since 1993, when the topic was debated in the 'Heathrow Debate' (DoH, 1993).

There is a historical divide between doctors and nurses that can create rivalries and prejudices. Anecdotal evidence suggests that some doctors regard nurses as 'lesser' people with inadequate training. Fortunately, this tends to be the view of older doctors, who will retire before partnership becomes a reality. Bower (1994) suggests that female general practitioners who are striving in a male-dominated profession are less willing to support the advanced role of nurses.

Nurses and doctors should be equal partners involved in the planning and management of patient care (Dowling et al., 1996). However, there is a positive disincentive to appoint a nurse rather than a general practitioner as a partner within a general practice as only a general practitioner partner attracts partnership payments and additional per capita payments. This reinforces the traditional models of primary care and is a clear barrier to progress (NHSE, 1996).

Parkinson (1996) reports on three nurse practitioners who successfully work in partnership with general practitioners. Although not financial partners, the nurses are involved in practice decisions and development. It is not unreasonable to expect to see more nurse–doctor partnerships in the future.

Radical changes in primary health care have been addressed by the DoH (1996b) in 'Choice and Opportunity – Primary Care: The Future'. The traditional structure of general practitioner partnerships is challenged by a suggestion of practice-based contracts that would embrace non-medical professionals, including nurses. Legislation to enable practices to pilot different types of contract is already in place, although nurse-led applications for pilot schemes were fewer in number than expected. Innovative practice nurses will rise to this challenge and prove that salaried partners are a viable option, nurses' skills complementing doctors'.

A call for nurses to forge partnerships with general practitioners was made at the 1997 RCN Congress, where the advantages to primary care development and health care were debated. The RCN was asked to consider the possibility of low-interest loans to enable nurses to enter a partnership (Practice Nurse, 1997), although no formal decision appeared to be given.

The need to obtain independent professional legal advice and indemnity is crucial in order to protect the nurse in this challenging position. Ten Wolverhampton general practitioners and ten practice nurses were canvassed in 1994 for their views on general practitioner–nurse partnerships (Edwards, 1995), the results being used during a seminar for community nurses to encourage debate on the future of partnerships. Nurses appeared more willing to embrace partnerships even if they did not see themselves as future partners. The results of the survey can be seen in Table 9.2.

Ideally, general practitioner–community nurse partnerships should be the future of general practice teams. In reality, workload (both paid employment and home/child care) and lack of finance to contribute to a partnership may inhibit many interested nurses from pursuing this course of action.

Table 9.2: Results of a questionnaire used to determine the views of nine general practitioners and eight practice nurses on partnerships (three non-responders)

General practitioners	Practice nurses
Advantages of general practitioner– practice nurse partnership	
Asset to practice	Improved decision-making
Motivated nurse	Lighten general practitioner workload
Financial gain for practice nurse	Financial gain
Joint care	Co-operation
Teamwork/co-operation	Greater autonomy
Improved clerical input/economy	Career prospects
Relieve doctor of on-call	Better patient care
	Female view on male-dominated practice
	More say in practice protocols
Disadvantages of general practitioner–practice nurse partnership	
Conflicting views	General practitioner threatened
Difficult decision-making	Financial input
Issues of responsibility	Needs full-time commitment
Disputes over profit-sharing	Reduced job mobility
Enough conflict with doctors!	Second best doctor
Legal issues	Legal issues
Nurse wanting to 'cover' herself	Unequal workload
FHSA reimbursement	Being on call
General practitioner feeling threatened	
Partnership issues	
Financial input? salaried?	

Integrated nursing

Integrated (community) nursing refers to combining the different skills, knowledge and expertise of a team of nurses to provide a comprehensive health care service that responds to the health needs of a defined community. This idea has developed in response to an acknowledgement of the inefficiency, fragmentation and overlap within community nursing service provision (Young, 1997).

Although the RCN is committed to the ideal of integrated nursing, few guidelines are offered on how to achieve it. Integrated nursing is not intended to be a cost-cutting exercise where fewer nurses do more work in a generic capacity, but to achieve improved, more significant and more accessible services to patients, with higher job satisfaction for nurses.

The success of primary health care depends on good team work, and although practice nurses may consider themselves part of the practice team, they rarely feel part of the wider community nursing team. Atkin and Lunt (1996) reported how general practitioners and purchasers both agreed that general practice should be the basis for teamworking, the roles of nursing staff being defined by 'skills' and 'expertise' rather than job title.

The role of the practice nurse varies greatly but often involves role overlap with district nurses and health visitors. This overlap can be managed constructively within an integrated team to maximize health care resources.

Shropshire has developed a framework for integrated nursing that can be adapted to individual team needs (Paterson, 1997). Two essential ingedients for this model are the need for good communication between team members and the motivation to develop the skills for team development.

The future

Community nurses and practice nurses are usually employed by different bodies, i.e. an NHS trust or general practitioner. There is a fear that direct employment by general practitioners may result in some nurses being forced back into the traditional handmaiden role. The political health policies that result in uncertainty about the future management of general practice are a complex subject and will not be discussed within this text.

There is a need to ensure that an open and effective communication system prevails in spite of different conditions of employment, the physical environment, arbitary divisions of labour and professional prejudice (Rowley, 1994). The expanding role of the practice nurse may create anxiety with regard to job losses for other primary health care colleagues. These fears must be allayed as each team member has valuable skills that are essential for comprehensive patient care. The emphasis must be on teamwork and not rivalry.

The role of each professional must be developed to meet the needs of the practice population. Teamwork should improve communication, prevent an overlap of services and lead to an improvement in patient care.

Traditionally, the general practitioner largely determined the service that the practice nurse offered to the practice population. This is changing. Some of the main changes in doctor–nurse–patient relationships are outlined in Box 9.10. Nurses are trained in a wide range of specialized skills and can offer a proactive approach to health. They are now in a position to advise the general practitioner.

Box 9.10: Changes in nurse–doctor relationships

Past
- The nurse was delegated tasks by the general practitioner
- The doctor instructed the nurse
- The patient was informed of his care
- The nurse was handmaiden to the doctor

Present
- The nurse directs patient care
- The doctor asks the nurse's advice
- There is negotiated/shared management
- The nurse is a professional equal

The prospect of a commissioning strategy for employing all primary health care nurses was reported by Atkin and Lunt (1995). Although it was recognized that practice nurses would continue to be employed by general practitioners, some purchasing authorities have attempted to gain greater managerial control over practice nurses.

Practice nurses have had a poorly defined role, a small proportion of nurses being employed for a specific role in the practice, such as health promotion, chronic disease management or treatment room tasks, and others undertaking a range of tasks and duties (Atkin and Lunt, 1995). The future of practice nursing involves a more specialized division of labour in which individual nurses have complementary skills to meet the needs of the practice population. Appropriate delegation and some skill mix is essential.

Most nurses surveyed by Atkin and Lunt (1995) considered practice nursing as a career, although a significant minority saw it as a job. This may be reflected in practice nurse interest in the changes in general practice as a whole. The former group will be the leaders of the future, whilst the latter group will undertake delegated tasks.

Research

Nurses must constantly be prepared to move into areas of practice that will maximize their healing role, and undertake research and evaluation to achieve the best possible health for patients and clients.

It is continually stressed that nurses should apply only evidence-based care. There is little published research by practice nurses, suggesting that the evidence base used may not always be appropriate to general practice.

The reader is urged to reflect on an area of practice of personal interest that might merit research (Figure 9.2 page 314). A prospective researcher can obtain initial advice on undertaking a project from the DHA primary care nurse adviser, although it is probably more helpful to undertake a research skills module through higher education.

Funding is available from several sources, including:

- scholarships, which are advertised regularly in the nursing press;
- DHA funding or part-funding of a module;
- an employer, if keen enough about the project;
- pharmaceutical funding. For example, a company selling medication for respiratory diseases, cardiovascular disease or diabetes may be willing to fund a research project in that area of health care. Pharmaceutical representatives will be able to advise on the amount of available funding, if any. Research projects do not have to be major works; it is the relevance to patient care that is important.

Accountability

Practice nurses should look critically at the work that general practitioners expect them to undertake. Does merely enhancing the general practitioner's income meet nurses' professional standards? Nurses must ensure that they receive the correct training for all aspects of their work, such as travel advice, health promotion, immunizations or cervical cytology. Case-studies describing various incidents relating to accountability are discussed by Jones (1996). These real scenarios highlight the difficulties that nurses encounter when overworked and undertrained. Every nurse must ensure that he or she does not put at risk the welfare of patients/clients. Regular updating to keep abreast of current policy in specific areas of practice is essential for all nurses.

The enhancement of nursing practice and the fulfilment of nursing potential demands a continuous review of professional activities

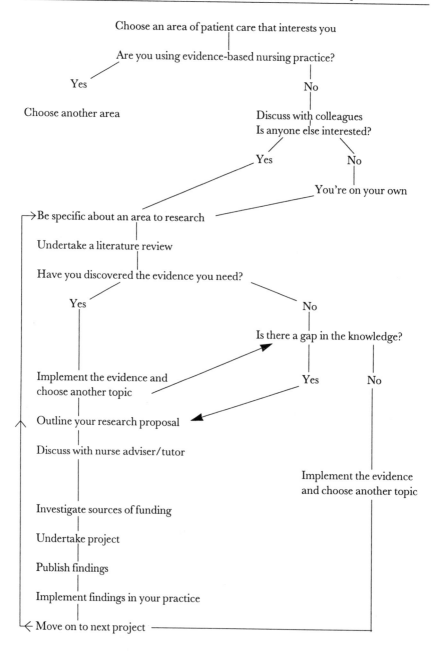

Figure 9.2: Undertaking a research project.

in order that the changing health needs of the population may be effectively met (Andrews, 1994). Nurse prescribing is a significant development among the many changes currently occurring within the profession.

Training

Community nurse education for the specialist practitioner qualification involves a common core of shared modules and specific specialized modules. It is hoped that this will promote collaboration and understanding between community nurses and reduce the professional rivalry between disciplines that is discussed by Atkin et al. (1993). It was suggested that as most practice nurses do not have this community qualification, they are likely to offer a poorer standard of service to the patient. This suggestion is an insult to practice nurses and must be challenged.

It is envisaged that graduates of this programme will become the care managers and team leaders of the future. Since 1999 all new community nurses are educated to degree level, eradicating some of the previous discrepancies between disciplines.

Increased finance for practice nurse training, with provision for locum cover, will lead to improved educational opportunities for nurses. Nurses must seize these opportunities to ensure that they are appropriately trained to meet their expanding roles. The DHA should be able to advise on the best way to access funding; some areas, via the nurse adviser, already actively encourage nurses to apply for funding.

New challenges

The future for nurse practitioners is exciting and challenging. General practitioner emergency services have developed throughout the UK to meet the need for out-of-hours medical care. The development and expansion of telephone helpline and triage services will help to reduce surgery visits and general practitioner call-outs, and increase the home management of minor illness. The nurse practitioner will have the skills to identify those patients who need to see a nurse or doctor.

Bowles (1995) suggested that nurse practitioners could set up independent practice as primary practitioners, consulting general practitioners as necessary. Is this any different from general practitioners consulting other specialists?

This is a realistic suggestion supported by Hunter (1996), who wrote that 'Fundholding general practitioners will be seeking a nursing service that is more responsive to practice needs. To do this, they will need independent nurses with extended roles and responsibilities who can work within the practice team.'

The political changes in 1997 will make radical change difficult, although not impossible. Once government strategies for primary health care have been more clearly defined, independent practice may be a realistic option for offering patients a choice of practitioner.

Summary

The nursing profession needs to identify the value of its role in general practice and develop not only the technical aspects of care, but also those which lie at the core of nursing and constitute the caring ethic.

Practice nurses make a valuable and major contribution to primary care, so professional development and career satisfaction are essential. Nurses must be encouraged to develop their role and autonomy within the primary health care team and to play a greater part in decision-making.

Patients and clients must not be misled, either inadvertently or intentionally; the role of the care-giver should be made clear to a recipient of care, whatever title a practitioner holds.

Resources for the NHS will always be finite, and it is essential to maximize the benefits for patients with the available resources. The NHSE (1996) promotes the development of partnerships in care, which includes increasing the role of non-medical staff in care provision. The primary health care team must adapt service provision to meet identified health needs and work together with shared philosophies and objectives. The need for continuing education and training, research and clinical audit emerged as key issues in the NHSE debate.

Nurses are continually developing their roles to provide more of the care previously provided by doctors. This role should not be regarded as a replacement for medical care but as a complementary role to the traditional medical model of care. Nurses who prefer to practise traditional clinical care skills rather than undertaking courses in higher education must not be devalued: high-quality individualized patient care is the mainstay of practice nursing. Nurses must practise at the level at which they are competent and confident. Grade/skill mix meets this need.

Higher education equips practice nurses to undertake research and clinical audit and offer evidence-based nursing care. Many nurses undertake valuable research and audit projects but do not publish their findings. This must be redressed to share knowledge and improve practice. Nurses will have the evidence with which to face any opposition by an employer when attempting to change practice. In a climate of increasing litigation, nurses must be sufficiently assertive to protect both their clients/patients and their own professional status.

The prospect of general practitioner–nurse partnerships should not be dismissed lightly. Limited NHS resources, a reduction in the number of general practitioner trainees and specialist training for nurses make the prospect of a general practitioner–nurse partnership a viable option for the future.

Key points:

1. Many practice nurses have extended roles.
2. The need to be trained for the role must not be underestimated.
3. Skill mix allows nurses to practise at their desired level.
4. Primary health care is more efficient when delivered by a team.

References

Andrews S (1994) Nurse prescribing. In Hunt G, Wainwright P (eds) Expanding the Role of the Nurse. London: Blackwell Science.

Atkin K, Lunt N (1995) Nurses in Practice. The Role of the Practice Nurse in Primary Health Care. Summary Report. University of York: Social Policy Research Unit.

Atkin K, Lunt N (1996) Negotiating the role of the nurse in general practice. Journal of Advanced Nursing 24: 498–505.

Atkin K, Lunt N, Parker G, Hirst M (1993) Nurses Count: A National Census of Practice Nurses. University of York: Social Policy Research Unit.

Bower H (1994) Practising for the future. Practice Nurse 8(5): 290–2.

Bowles A (1995) Independent growth. Practice Nurse 8(12): 686–91.

Butterworth CA, Faugier J (1993) Cited in National Health Service Executive (1996) Clinical Supervision – a Resource Pack for Practice Nurses. London: NHSE.

Castledine G (1995) Defining specialist nursing. British Journal of Nursing 4(5): 264–5.

Cook R, Leech F (1996) Clinical supervision. Primary Health Care 6(8): 12–13.

Cooper A (1997) Making skill mix work. Practice Nurse 13(9): 521–2.

Department of Health (1986) Neighbourhood Nursing – A Focus for Care. Report of the Community Nursing Review (Cumberlege Report). London: HMSO.

Department of Health (1989) DOH Report of the Advisory Group on Nurse Prescribing (Crown Report). London: HMSO.

Department of Health (1993) The Challenges for Nursing and Midwifery in the 21st Century – a Report on the Heathrow Debate. London: HMSO.

Department of Health (1996a) Primary Care: Delivering the future London: HMSO.

Department of Health (1996b) Choice and Opportunity – Primary Care: The Future. London: HMSO.

Dowling S, Martin R, Skidmore P, Doyal L, Cameron A, Lloyd S (1996) Nurses taking on junior doctors' work: a confusion of accountability. British Medical Journal (312): 1211–14.

Edwards M (1995) The future of practice nurse/GP partnerships. Practice Nursing 6(10): 36–8.

Elcock K (1996) Consultant nurse: an appropriate title for the advanced nurse practitioner? British Journal of Nursing 5(22): 1376–81.

English National Board for Nursing, Midwifery and Health Visiting (1990) The Challenge of Primary Health Care in the 1990's: A Review of Education and Training for Practice Nurses (Damant Report). London: ENB.

Fairfield H (1996) NVQ training in general practice. Primary Health Care 6(9): 14–16.

Fawcett Henesy A, West P (1995) Nurse practitioners: the South Thames Regional Authority experience. Nursing Times 91(12): 40–1.

General Medical Council (1995) Good Medical Practice. Duties of a Doctor. Guidance from the General Medical Council. London: GMC.

Greenfield S, Stilwell B, Drury M (1987) Practice nurses: social and occupational characteristics. Journal of the Royal College of General Practitioners 37: 341–7.

Hunter P (1996) Is this the next step for nursing? Practice Nurse 11(3): 174–6.

Jones M (1996) Accountability in Practice: A Guide to Professional Responsibility for Nurses in General Practice. Dinton: Quay Books.

Jones M, Gough P (1997) Nurse prescribing – why has it taken so long? Nursing Standard 11(20): 39–42.

Marsh GN, Dawes ML (1995) Establishing a minor illness nurse in a busy general practice. British Medical Journal 310: 778–80.

National Health Service Executive (1996) Primary Care: The Future. London: NHSE.

Parkinson C (1996) So you want to be a ... GP practice partner. Community Nurse 2(4): 51.

Paterson J (1997) Stage is set for new nurse teams. Practice Nurse 14(7): 425–8.

Practice Nurse (1997) Call for partnerships with GPs. Practice Nurse 13(10): 579.

Rashid A, Watts A, Lenehan C, Haslam D (1996) Skill-mix in primary care: sharing clinical workload and understanding professional roles. British Journal of General Practice 46(412): 639–40.

Rees M, Kinnersley P (1996) Nurse-led management of minor illness in a GP surgery. Nursing Times 92(6): 32–3.

Richardson G, Maynard A (1995) Fewer Doctors? More Nurses? A Review of the Knowledge Base of Doctor–Nurse Substitution. York: University of York.

Ross FM, Bowe PJ, Sibbald BS (1994) Practice nurses: characteristics, workload and training needs. British Journal of General Practice 44: 15–18.

Rowley E (1994) The role of the practice nurse. In Hunt G, Wainwright P (eds) Expanding the Role of the Nurse. London: Blackwell Science.

Royal College of Nursing (1995) RCN Factsheet: Nurse Prescribing. London: RCN.

Royal College of Nursing (1997a) Nurse Practitioners: Your Questions Answered. London: RCN.

Royal College of Nursing (1997b) Practice Nursing and Skill Mix. Leaflet No. 42. London: RCN.

Smith M (1993) Skill mix in general practice. Practice Nursing 16 Nov – 12 Dec: 21.

Stilwell B (1984) The nurse in practice. Nursing Mirror 158(21): 17–19.

Stilwell B (1988) The origins and development of the nurse practitioner. In Bowling A, Stilwell B (eds) The Nurse in Family Practice. London: Scutari Press.

Stilwell B (1991) The rise of the practice nurse. Nursing Times 87(24): 26–7.

Stilwell B, Greenfield S, Drury M, Hull FM (1987) A nurse practitioner in general practice: working style and pattern of consultation. Journal of the Royal College of General Practitioners 37: 154–7.

Thomson R (1996) Nurses who dispense post-coital contraception. Community Nurse 1(12): 27–8.

United Kingdom Central Council for Nursing, Midwifery and Health Visitors (1991) Report on Proposals for the Future of Community Education and Practice. London: UKCC.

United Kingdom Central Council for Nursing, Midwifery and Health Visiting (1992a) The Scope of Professional Practice. London: UKCC.

United Kingdom Central Council for Nursing, Midwifery and Health Visiting (1992b) Standards for the Administration of Medicines. London: UKCC.

United Kingdom Central Council for Nursing, Midwifery and Health Visiting (1992c) Code of Professional Conduct. London: UKCC.

United Kingdom Central Council for Nursing, Midwifery and Health Visiting (1993) Final Report on the Future of Professional Education and Practice. London: UKCC.

United Kingdom Central Council for Nursing, Midwifery and Health Visiting (1994a) The Future of Professional Practice – the Council's Standards for Education and Practice Following Registration. London: UKCC.

United Kingdom Central Council for Nursing, Midwifery and Health Visiting (1994b) Registrar's Letter No. 20. London: UKCC.

United Kingdom Central Council for Nursing, Midwifery and Health Visiting (1996) Registrar's Letter No. 15. London: UKCC.

United Kingdom Central Council for Nursing, Midwifery and Health Visiting (1997) Register. 19:5. London: UKCC.

Whitehead M (1988) The Health Divide. London: Penguin.

Winstanley F (1996) Evaluation on site. Primary Health Care 6(1): 11–12.

Young L (1997) Integrated nursing teams. Primary Health Care 7(6): 8, 10.

Useful addresses

Further information about courses leading to recordable or specialist qualifications can be obtained from the following:

English National Board for Nursing, Midwifery and Health Visiting
Victory House,
170 Tottenham Court Road,
London W1P OHA

Tel: 0171-388 3131

Tel: 0171-388 3131
National Board for Nursing, Midwifery and Health Visiting for Northern Ireland
Centre House,
70 Chichester Street,
Belfast BT1 4JE
Tel: (01233) 238152

National Board for Nursing, Midwifery and Health Visiting for Scotland
22 Queen Street,
Edinburgh EH2 1NT
Tel: 0131-226 7371

Welsh National Board for Nursing, Midwifery and Health Visiting
Floor 13,
Pearl Assurance House,
Greyfriars Road,
Cardiff CF1 3AG
Tel: (01222) 395535

Index